A new and easy method of cookery. Treating, I. Of gravies, soups, broths, ... II. Of fish, and their sauces. ... VI. Of made wines, distilling and brewing, ... By Elizabeth Cleland. ... The second edition.

Elizabeth Cleland

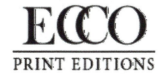

ECCO
PRINT EDITIONS

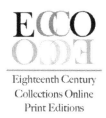

Eighteenth Century
Collections Online
Print Editions

Gale ECCO Print Editions

Relive history with *Eighteenth Century Collections Online*, now available in print for the independent historian and collector. This series includes the most significant English-language and foreign-language works printed in Great Britain during the eighteenth century, and is organized in seven different subject areas including literature and language; medicine, science, and technology; and religion and philosophy. The collection also includes thousands of important works from the Americas.

The eighteenth century has been called "The Age of Enlightenment." It was a period of rapid advance in print culture and publishing, in world exploration, and in the rapid growth of science and technology – all of which had a profound impact on the political and cultural landscape. At the end of the century the American Revolution, French Revolution and Industrial Revolution, perhaps three of the most significant events in modern history, set in motion developments that eventually dominated world political, economic, and social life.

In a groundbreaking effort, Gale initiated a revolution of its own: digitization of epic proportions to preserve these invaluable works in the largest online archive of its kind. Contributions from major world libraries constitute over 175,000 original printed works. Scanned images of the actual pages, rather than transcriptions, recreate the works *as they first appeared.*

Now for the first time, these high-quality digital scans of original works are available via print-on-demand, making them readily accessible to libraries, students, independent scholars, and readers of all ages.

For our initial release we have created seven robust collections to form one the world's most comprehensive catalogs of 18th century works.

Initial Gale ECCO Print Editions collections include:

History and Geography
Rich in titles on English life and social history, this collection spans the world as it was known to eighteenth-century historians and explorers. Titles include a wealth of travel accounts and diaries, histories of nations from throughout the world, and maps and charts of a world that was still being discovered. Students of the War of American Independence will find fascinating accounts from the British side of conflict.

Social Science

Delve into what it was like to live during the eighteenth century by reading the first-hand accounts of everyday people, including city dwellers and farmers, businessmen and bankers, artisans and merchants, artists and their patrons, politicians and their constituents. Original texts make the American, French, and Industrial revolutions vividly contemporary.

Medicine, Science and Technology

Medical theory and practice of the 1700s developed rapidly, as is evidenced by the extensive collection, which includes descriptions of diseases, their conditions, and treatments. Books on science and technology, agriculture, military technology, natural philosophy, even cookbooks, are all contained here.

Literature and Language

Western literary study flows out of eighteenth-century works by Alexander Pope, Daniel Defoe, Henry Fielding, Frances Burney, Denis Diderot, Johann Gottfried Herder, Johann Wolfgang von Goethe, and others. Experience the birth of the modern novel, or compare the development of language using dictionaries and grammar discourses.

Religion and Philosophy

The Age of Enlightenment profoundly enriched religious and philosophical understanding and continues to influence present-day thinking. Works collected here include masterpieces by David Hume, Immanuel Kant, and Jean-Jacques Rousseau, as well as religious sermons and moral debates on the issues of the day, such as the slave trade. The Age of Reason saw conflict between Protestantism and Catholicism transformed into one between faith and logic -- a debate that continues in the twenty-first century.

Law and Reference

This collection reveals the history of English common law and Empire law in a vastly changing world of British expansion. Dominating the legal field is the *Commentaries of the Law of England* by Sir William Blackstone, which first appeared in 1765. Reference works such as almanacs and catalogues continue to educate us by revealing the day-to-day workings of society.

Fine Arts

The eighteenth-century fascination with Greek and Roman antiquity followed the systematic excavation of the ruins at Pompeii and Herculaneum in southern Italy; and after 1750 a neoclassical style dominated all artistic fields. The titles here trace developments in mostly English-language works on painting, sculpture, architecture, music, theater, and other disciplines. Instructional works on musical instruments, catalogs of art objects, comic operas, and more are also included.

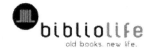

The BiblioLife Network

This project was made possible in part by the BiblioLife Network (BLN), a project aimed at addressing some of the huge challenges facing book preservationists around the world. The BLN includes libraries, library networks, archives, subject matter experts, online communities and library service providers. We believe every book ever published should be available as a high-quality print reproduction; printed on-demand anywhere in the world. This insures the ongoing accessibility of the content and helps generate sustainable revenue for the libraries and organizations that work to preserve these important materials.

The following book is in the "public domain" and represents an authentic reproduction of the text as printed by the original publisher. While we have attempted to accurately maintain the integrity of the original work, there are sometimes problems with the original work or the micro-film from which the books were digitized. This can result in minor errors in reproduction. Possible imperfections include missing and blurred pages, poor pictures, markings and other reproduction issues beyond our control. Because this work is culturally important, we have made it available as part of our commitment to protecting, preserving, and promoting the world's literature.

GUIDE TO FOLD-OUTS MAPS and OVERSIZED IMAGES

The book you are reading was digitized from microfilm captured over the past thirty to forty years. Years after the creation of the original microfilm, the book was converted to digital files and made available in an online database.

In an online database, page images do not need to conform to the size restrictions found in a printed book. When converting these images back into a printed bound book, the page sizes are standardized in ways that maintain the detail of the original. For large images, such as fold-out maps, the original page image is split into two or more pages

Guidelines used to determine how to split the page image follows:

• Some images are split vertically; large images require vertical and horizontal splits.
• For horizontal splits, the content is split left to right.
• For vertical splits, the content is split from top to bottom.
• For both vertical and horizontal splits, the image is processed from top left to bottom right.

A
NEW AND EASY
METHOD
OF
COOKERY.

TREATING,

I. Of GRAVIES, SOUPS, BROTHS, &c.

II. Of F I S H, and their SAUCES.

III. To Pot and Make HAMS, &c.

IV. Of PIES, PASTIES, &c.

V. Of PICKLING and PRESERVING.

VI. Of Made WINES, DISTILLING and BREWING, &c.

TO WHICH ARE ADDED,

By Way of APPENDIX,

Fifty-Three NEW and USEFUL RECEIPTS, and DIRECTIONS for CARVING.

By ELIZABETH CLELAND.

Chiefly intended for the Benefit of the Young LADIES *who attend Her* SCHOOL.

The SECOND EDITION.

E D I N B U R G H:
Printed by C. WRIGHT and COMPANY: And fold at their Printing-houfe in *Craig's Clofe,* and by the Bookfellers in Town.
M.DCC.LIX

THE CONTENTS.

CHAP. I.

Of Gravies, Soups, Broths and Pottages.

CHAP. II.

Of dressing all Kinds of Fish, and their Sauces.

a　To

CONTENTS.

CHAP.

CONTENTS.

CHAP. III.

To pot and make Hams, &c.

CONTENTS.

CHAP.

CONTENTS.
CHAP. IV.
To make Pies and Pasties, &c.

To

CONTENTS.

A

CONTENTS.

Maids

CONTENTS.

Macaroons

CONTENTS.

CHAP. V.

Of Pickling, and Preferving, &c.

CONTENTS:

CHAP VI.

Of made Wines, &c.

APPEN.

APPENDIX.

A

A
NEW and EASY
METHOD of COOKERY.

+++

CHAP I.

Of GRAVIES, SOUPS, BROTHS, and POTTAGES.

+++

To make a strong Broth for Soups or Sauces.

TAKE a Hough of Beef, or any coarse Piece, and set it over the Fire, in four *English* Gallons of Water, skim it clean, season it with Salt, whole black and *Jamaica* Pepper, Mace, Cloves, a Bunch of sweet Herbs, and six or seven Onions; boil it on a very slow Fire, for four Hours, then strain it, and keep it for Use.

To make brown Gravy for Soups.

CUT three or four Pounds of coarse Beef in thin Slices, put it in a Frying-Pan, with a very little Piece of Butter, a sliced Carot and Turnip, and Onions,

A   with

with a Bunch of fweet Herbs ; **cover it clofe, put it
on a very flow Fire, fry it brown, but don't burn it;**
then put to it fome good Broth, then boil all together
very well, and keep it for Soups or Sauces ; feafon it
with Pepper, Salt, *Jamaica* Pepper and Cloves.

White Gravy for Soups or Sauces.

TAKE a Knuckle of Veal, and boil it in fix *En-glifh* Quarts of Water, till it is in Strings, then ftrain
it ; but when it is half boiled, put in whole Mace,
Pepper, Cloves and Salt, fo keep it for Ufe. You
make Gravy of Mutton the fame Way.

A good Stock for Fifh Soups.

PREPARE Scate Flounders and Eels, lay them in a
broad Gravy Pan, with a Sprig of Thyme, Parfley and
Onions, feafon them with Pepper, Salt, Cloves and
Mace, then pour in as much Water as will cover them,
boil them on a very flow Fire for an Hour, then ftrain
it off. if it is for brown Soup or Sauces, put in the
Skins of the Onions, and a brown Cruft of Bread, with
dried Mufhrooms ; keep the Gravy Pan clofs covered.

A Vermicelli Soup.

TAKE three *Englifh* Quarts of good Broth, put in
it two Ounces of Vermicelli, and a Bit of lean Bacon,
ftuffed with Cloves, put two Chickens or a boiled Fowl
in it : You may make Rice Soup the fame Way, but
boil the Rice firft in Water, then in Broth ; half an
Hour boils the Vermicelli.

To make a Craw-fifh or Lobfter Soup.

LET your Stock be as in Page firft, take as many as
will fill your Difh, then take out the Sand-bags out of

the

the **Tails**, and all the woolly Parts that are about them; put them in a Sauce-pan with your Soup, with Crumbs of **Bread**, and a little Butter, peel an Onion, ſtuff it with Cloves, and boil all the Shells in the Fiſh Stock, before you put in the Tail, and take them out when they are well boiled; ſtrain your Stock before you put in the Fiſh or any Seaſoning.

A Veal Soup with Barley.

YOUR Stock muſt be with a Fowl, and a Knuckle of Veal, ſeaſoned only with Mace, then ſtrain all off; put in half a Pound of fine Barley, boil it an Hour; ſeaſon it with Salt, put the Fowl in the Middle, and juſt as you ſerve it up, put in chopped Parſley.

A green Peaſe Soup.

TAKE a Peck of young green Peaſe, put them in a Stew Pot, cover them with Water, put in a little Thyme, Parſley, Onion, Pepper, Salt, and a good Lump of Butter; then cover them, and let them ſtew a while; then cut four Cabbage Lettices in Quarters, with ſix Cucumbers pared and ſliced, and a Handful of Purſlain; put them in the Soup with a Piece of Butter, and more ſeaſoning; then fill your Pan with Water; the Soup will take Stewing two Hours, if the Liquor is too much waſted away in that Time, add a little more boiling Water to it, you may put Slices of fried Bacon in the Diſh, or a roaſted Fowl if you pleaſe.

A brown Pottage Royal.

SET a Gallon of ſtrong Broth over the Fire, with two ſhivered Palates, Cocks Combs, Lambs Stones ſliced, with forc'd meat Balls, a Pint of Gravy, two Handfuls of Spinage and young Lettice minced, boil theſe together with a Duck, the Leg and Wing being

being broke, and the Bones pulled out, and the Breaſt flaſhed, and browned in a Pan of Fat; then put the Pottage in a Diſh, and the Duck in the Middle; lay about it a little Vermicelli, boiled up in ſome ſtrong Broth, with ſavoury Forc'd-Meat Balls, and Sweet Breads; boil the Duck in the Broth for half an Hour before you diſh it.

Rice Soup.

TAKE a Quarter of a Pound of Rice, waſh it, boil it in Veal Broth till very tender, with a little Mace and a young Fowl; ſkim it very clean, and ſeaſon it with Salt to your Taſte; then ſtir in half a Pound of Butter, and a Mutchkin of Cream boiled up; then ſtir it in the Soup; ſerve it up with the Fowl.

Barley Pottage.

LAY a Pound of fine Barley to ſteep in two Chopins of Cream, ſome Salt, Mace and Cinnamon, when it is thick, ſweeten it to your Taſte.

A Pottage, forc'd Pigeons with Onions.

WASH and blanch them, take a Piece of Veal, a little Suet, pound them, and ſeaſon it with Pepper, Salt, Nutmeg, Lemon-peel, ſweet Herbs, Chives, Parſley and Muſhrooms, all chopped ſmall; mix all together with Crumbs of Bread, and as many raw Eggs as will wet it; put it in your Pigeons, and ſtop their Vents; ſet them to boil in good Broth, take ſmall Onions, boil them and drain them, then put them to the Pigeons; take the Cruſts of fine Bread in ſome of the Broth, and put them in the Diſh under the Pigeons, and pour the Pottage on them.

To make *Plumb Broth.*

TAKE a good Hough of Beef, and a Knuckle of Veal, put it in the Pot with fix *Scots* Pints of Water, boil it on a flow Fire; take up the Veal before it is too much, but boil the Beef to pieces; if the Broth is too ftiff, put in a Pint of boiling Water, put in the Crumbs of two Penny Loaves, two Pounds of Currants wafhed clean, two of Raifins ftoned, one of Prunes, let all boil till they fwell; feafon it with Salt, Cloves, Mace, and Nutmeg, ftrain the Broth before you put in the Fruit.

To make *Spring Soup.*

TAKE twelve Lettices, cut them in Slices and put them into ftrong Broth, get fix green Cucumbers, pare them, and cut out the Cores, cut them into little Bits, and fcald them in boiling Water, and put them into your Broth, let them boil very tender, with a Mutchkin of young Peafe and fome Crumbs of Bread.

Pottage of Chervil the Dutch *Way.*

PUT into eight Chopins of good Broth a Knuckle of Veal, cut in Pieces the Bignefs of an Egg, don't let it boil too faft, but keep it fkim'd; feafon it with Pepper, Salt, Cloves and Mace, a Quarter of an Hour before you difh it; put in a good deal of Chervil chopp'd fmall, fome Forc'd-meat Balls, and fome Crumbs of Bread; let them boil well before you put them in, but not too much; fo difh it.

Jelly Broth for confumptive Perfons.

GET a Joint of Mutton, a Capon, a Fillet of Veal, put them in an Earthen Can clofe ftopt, with three

Quarts of Water; then put the Can in a Pot of Water, and when all the Flesh is boil'd to Rags strain it off for Use.

To make Soup de Sante the French *Way*.

BOIL a Hough of Beef to Tavers on a very slow Fire; skim it, and when there is only what will fill your Dish, strain it; take three Pounds of Beef, cut in thin Slices, put it in a Pan with sliced Onions, Carots and Turnips in it, and a little Bit of Butter, till the Meat is brown, and the Pan dry; then pour your Soup on it, boil it an Hour, skim it and strain it; then get Chervil, Sorrel, Endive, Sellery, and Cabbage Lettices; cut them, but not too small, half boil them in Water, drain them, then put them in a closs Goblet with your Soup, boil them till the Herbs are tender, season it with an Onion stuffed with Cloves, Pepper and Salt, put in the Dish a boiled Knuckle of Veal, or a Fowl, two *French* Rolls, the Crust only, or toasted Bread.

To make a Summer Pottage.

TAKE a Hough of Beef, a Scrag of Mutton or Veal, chop them, and boil them gently in a sufficient Quantity of Water for six Hours, being covered close; then put in four Onions, and whole Pepper; when the Meat is boiled to Rags, strain it, put in Cloves, Mace, and a Faggot of sweet Herbs, with Sorrel, Beets, Endive and Spinage, of each a Handful, shred grosly, boil it till they are tender, put it in the Dish with roasted Pigeons, or Ducks, in the Middle of it, and small Slices of fried Bacon, toasted Bread cut in Dice, Sausages cut in little Bits; in the Time of Asparagus, cut into Pieces the green Part, and boil them in it.

To make Meagre Broth for Soups with Herbs.

SET on the Fire a Kettle of Water, put in it some Crusts of Bread, and all Sorts of Herbs, green Beets, Sellery, Endive, Lettice, Sorrel, green Onions, Parsley, Chervil, with a good Piece of Butter, and a Bunch of sweet Herbs, boil it for an Hour and a Half, then strain it off; this will serve to make Artichoke or Asparagus, or *Soup de sante* with Herbs; season it with Salt, Pepper, Cloves, *Jamaica* Pepper; cut the Herbs grossly, and it will be a very good Soup, boiling a good Lump of Butter with the Herbs, putting toasted Bread in the Dish; but take out the Bulk of the sweet Herbs.

To make Scots *Barley* Broth.

BOIL a Hough of Beef in eight Pints of Water, and a Pound of Barley on a slow Fire; let it boil to four Pints; then put in Onions, Pepper, Salt and Raisins if you like them, or you may put in Greens and Leeks.

A Calf's Head Soup.

TAKE a Calf's Head, stew it tender; then strain off the Liquor, and put in a Bunch of sweet Herbs, Onions, Salt, Pepper, Mace, and some fine Barley, boil it till the Barley and Head is done; then serve it with the Head in the Middle.

To make Mutton Broth.

TAKE about six Pounds of Mutton, boil it in three *Scots* Pints of Water, with sweet Herbs, Onions, two or three Turnips, a Quarter of a Pound of fine Barley or Rice, Salt and Pepper; a little before you take it up, put in it a Handful of chopped Parsley.

To make another Barley Broth.

TAKE a Neck and Breast of Mutton, cut it to Pieces, put as much Water as will cover it; when it boils skim it; put in Barley, diced Carots, Turnips, Onions, a Faggot of Thyme and Parsley, Pepper and Salt, stove all well together; you may put in a Sheep's Head, but first singe and scrape it, and soak it well in Water; to make this green, put Beet Leaves, Brocoli, and green Onions, all shred small.

A Purslain Soup.

WHEN your Purslain is young, cut the Sprigs off, but keep their whole Length; boil them in a Stew-pan, with some Pease-soup, and small Onions, when your Purslain is boiled in good Broth, put a Crust of Bread soaked in Broth in the Dish, then pour your Soup on it with the Purslain; season it to your Taste.

A Cucumber Soup.

PARE and slice them, not very thin, stew them in a little Butter, and put them in strong Broth, seasoned with Pepper, Salt and Onions, so serve them up.

To make Soup Meagre.

BOIL two or three Pounds of coarse Beef in eight Chopins of Water, boil it to four; then strain it off; then fry Slices of Carots, Turnips and Onions, in clarified Butter; drain them very well, put them in with Sorrel, Beets, Purslain, Endive, Sellery, Cabbage-Lettice, of each a Handful; cut them grosly, and put them all in the Soup, with Crusts of Bread, a Bunch of Parsley, green Onions and Thyme; season it with Pepper

per, Cloves and Salt; after you put in your Herbs
and Greens, boil them till the Roots are enough; boil
the Roots and Sellery in it before you put in the
rest.

An Eel Soup.

TAKE Eels according to the Quantity of Soup you
would have, a Pound of Eels will make a Mutchkin of
Soup; to every Pound of Eels add a Chopin of Water,
a Crust of Bread, two or three Blades of Mace, whole
Pepper, an Onion, and a Faggot of sweet Herbs, cover them closs, and let them boil till Half the Liquor is
wasted; then strain it, and put Toasts of Bread cut in
Dice in the Dish, then pour on your Soup; you may
put Forc'd meat Balls made of Fish, or Bread, in it.

An Almond Soup.

YOUR Stock must be of Veal, blanch and beat a
Pound of *Jordan* Almonds very fine, with the Yolks of
six hard Eggs, putting a little cold Broth in as you
pound them, then put in as much Broth as will fill the
Dish, put it on the Fire, stir it often, then strain it
off, and put in two small Chickens, and some Slices
of fine Bread, season it with white Pepper, Mace and
Salt, send it up hot.

Onion Soup.

TAKE Half a Pound of Butter, put it in a Stew-
pan on the Fire, and boil it till it has done making a
Noise, then take ten Onions, pared and cut small,
throw them in the Butter, and let them fry a while,
then shake in a little Flour, keep it stirring all the
while, and let them do a little longer; then pour in
three Mutchkins of boiling Water, stir them round, cut
small the upper Crust of the stalest Penny Loaf you
have, and put in it, season it with Pepper and Salt, let

it boil ten Minutes, take it off the Fire, beat the Yolks of two Eggs with Salt, a Spoonful of Vinegar, mix them, then ſtir it into the Soup; mix it well and diſh it.

A general Cullis for Fiſh.

WASH and ſcale ſome Carps, and cut them in Bits, put ſome Butter in a Pan, and place a good deal of Slices of Onions, and the Bill of the Carp in it, put it on a ſlow Fire, and when the Onions ſtick to the Bottom, put in ſome Peaſe Soup; put in a Sprig of Thyme, Parſley, Chives, Pepper, Cloves, and Mace, you may put in it a Clove of Rockambole or Garlick, if you like it; put a Lump of Butter into another Stew-pan, and put it on the Fire, with as much Flour as will thicken it; ſtir it till it is a light brown, then put a little of the Carp Liquor in by Degrees, keeping it ſtirring all the Time; then pour all together with Anchovies, dry Muſhrooms, and Lemon peel, with the Juice of it, and two Gills of white Wine; you may put in Gravy if you pleaſe. This Cullis will do for any Fiſh Soup or Cullis; you may make any Fiſh the ſame Way.

A Veal Cullis.

PUT in a Stew pan a Piece of Butter, then cut Slices of Veal and lay them in it, with ſome Slices of a Carot, Turnip and Onions, and Slices of Ham if you like it; cover it cloſs, and when the Veal is brown take it out, and ſhake into your Pan a little Flour, keep it ſtirring with a Spoon till the Flour is brown; then put in ſome Broth by Degrees, keep it ſtewing all the while; if you have no Broth put in Water, put in as much as you will want, then put in the Veal with a Bunch of ſweet Herbs, whole Pepper, Mace, Onion ſtuffed with Cloves, and ſome Lemon-peel, let it ſtew well

on

on a flow Fire, put in a Gill of white Wine, and when it is a good Brown, and the Veal well boiled in it, ftrain it off; take off all the Fat, and you may ufe it with all Sorts of Entries.

Green Cullis for Soups or Sauces.

LET green Peafe be done without Liquor, then take Parfley, Spinage and green Onions, of each a Handful; blanch them, fqueeze them well, and pound them, put in fome Broth, with a Bit of Ham, an O-nion ftuffed with Cloves, fome Slices of Veal, a Bunch of fweet Herbs, your Peafe and Veal muft be ftewed before you put in the Broth; and when clammy, put in the Broth and Juice of the Herbs, when all ftews a while, take out the Meat, and pound the Peafe, and then mix all together; feafon it with Pepper, Salt, and Mace, put in more green Parfley and green Oni-ons, boil all, and when boil'd ftrain it, it will ferve in all green Soups and Sauces.

To make a brown Soup.

PUT in your Broth Pot a Hough of Beef, but firft cut fome of the beft Pieces in thin Slices, fkim your Pot, and let it boil very flow, fry your Steaks a little brown, and when your Broth is boiled, put it to your Steaks, with a little fweet Herbs, two or three whole Onions, whole Black, and Clove Pepper and Cloves, before you put in your Ingredients, fkim off all the Fat, you may put in Vermicelli in your Difh, or Sel-lery with toafted Bread, boil your Vermicelli and Sellery before you put it in your Soup; ftrain your Soup before you put it to your fried Collops, put in your Broth by Degrees.

To make a white Soup.

BOIL a hind Leg of Lamb, Mutton or Veal, in Rags, then fkim off all the Fat, feafon it with Pepper,

Cloves

Cloves and Mace, (they muſt be all whole) two or three whole Onions, and a Bunch of ſweet Herbs; you may either whiten it with pounded Almonds or ſweet Cream; ſtrain it and ſalt it to your Taſte, ſend the Shank in it to the Table.

To make Peaſe Soup.

BOIL a Hough of Beef, with a Pound and a half of Peaſe, till they are all diſſolved, then ſtrain it and put in it whole Onions and Spice, ſalt it to your Taſte, brown ſome Butter and Flour and mix with it: You may put boil'd Sellery cut in Dice in it, if you pleaſe. Take the whole Onions always out of every Thing, before it goes to the Table put Spearmint in it.

To make Onion Soup.

TAKE ſome of the Broth of a Hough of Beef, and boil in it a Dozen large Onions cut in Slices, with black and *Jamaca* Pepper, Salt, and a Bunch of ſweet Herbs; thicken it with brown'd Butter and Flour and Crumbs of Bread: Take out your Herbs before it goes to the Table; let there be ſome ſmall whole Onions boil'd in it.

Aſparagus Soup.

TAKE ſome of the Broth of a Hough of Beef, and green it with the Juice of Spinage, cut half a Hundred of Aſparagus, half an Inch long, and boil them in it, with black and *Jamaica* Pepper, an Onion ſtuffed with Cloves, and a Bunch of ſweet Herbs; thicken it with Flour and Butter, boil it well after you put in the Butter and Flour.

To make Hodge-podge.

BOIL a Neck and Breaſt of Mutton in three Quarts of Water, ſkim it well, then put in Turnips and Carots cut in Dice; if they are old, boil them in Water firſt; when it is almoſt boil'd put in ſome Crumbs of Bread, two Onions, and a Chopin of green Peaſe, thicken it with brown'd Butter and Flour, put in it a brown'd Cruſt of Bread, Pepper and Salt; you may put in Sellery or Endive if you pleaſe; Brocoli or Aſparagus is very good in it, when you can't get Peaſe; take out the Cruſt of Bread before you ſend it to Table.

To make a green Peaſe Soup.

BOIL a Peck of Peaſe into two Quarts of Water till they are all in Smaſh, keep out a Mutchkin of the youngeſt, put them in a little before you diſh them; ſtrain and rub your Peaſe thro' a Search, then put it on the Fire again, and put a little Juice of Spinage in it, and a little Spearmint, Pepper and Salt to your Taſte, Half a Pound of Butter work'd in Flour, then your green Peaſe: Let it boil till you think it thick enough, and then ſerve it up. If you have a Mind to have it rich, inſtead of Water, put the Broth of a Hough of Beef, with a good white Gravy in it.

A very good Peaſe Soup.

BOIL three Pounds of lean Beef in eight Chopins of Water, and three Pound of Peaſe, till the Meat is all in Rags, then put in two or three Anchovies, a Faggot of Thyme, Spearmint, Parſley, and Ginger, Pepper, Salt and Cloves, with ſome Onions, then boil it for a while, and ſtrain it off in a clean Pan, then give it another Boil, ſtirring in it a good Piece of Butter. Fry ſome Forc'd meat Balls, Bacon cut in thin Slices, and

Bread

Bread cut in Dice, with Spinage boil'd green and chopped small, with a Bit of Butter and Salt, and roll'd in Balls: Put all in the Dish, and pour the Soup boiling hot over them.

To make a Pottage the French Way.

TAKE hard Lettices, Sorrel, Chervil, Beets and Spinage, of each a like Quantity, or any other Herbs you like, as much as a Half Peck will hold pressed down, pick, wash and drain them, put them in a Pot with a Pound of fresh Butter, and set them over the Fire, and, as the Butter melts, stir them down in it till they are as low as the Butter, then put in some Water, season it with Pepper, Cloves and Salt, put in a Crust of Bread, and some Chives, and when it is boil'd, take out the Bread, and thicken it with the Yolks of three or four Eggs, take Care they don't curdle, beat them well, put Toasts of Bread in the Dish with it.

To make Pottage of Chopped Herbs.

MINCE, very fine, Spinage, Chives, Parsley, Marigold-flowers, Succory, Strawberry and Violet Leaves, stamp them with Oat-meal in a Bowl, put chopped Greens in with it: you may either put Broth or Water to them, if Water, boil a good Piece of Butter in it; put Sipets in the Dish, and pour it over them.

A Fish Broth.

CUT Carots, Turnips and Onions, in thin Slices, put them into a Stew-Pan with a Lump of Butter, when they are brown put to them some Fish Broth, made of either Carps, Eels, Haddocks or Scate; then put in Parsley, Thyme, Chives, and some dry Mushrooms, season it with Pepper, Salt and Cloves, boil it an Hour with a Crust of Bread in it.

An

An Oifter Soup.

TAKE a Chopin of Oifters, wafh them clean in their own Liquor, then ftrain the Liquor, put to it two Gills of Water and one Gill of white Wine, a Sprig of Thyme and Parfley, a Shalot, a Bit of Lemon-peel, a few Cloves, a Blade of Mace, and fome whole Pepper, let them ftew gently for a little ; put a Quarter of a Pound of Butter into a Pan, flour it well, then let it fry till it has done hiffing, keep it ftirring ; then take the Oifters and dry them in a Cloth, and flour them, put them in the boiling Butter, and fry them till they are plump, then put in their own Liquor, with three Mutchkins of ftrong Broth, keep it ftirring all the Time : If your Soup is not brown, you may put Toafts in the Difh cut in Dice, and a *French* Loaf toafted.

To make Calves-feet Broth.

BOIL the Feet in juft as much Water as will make a good Jelly, then ftrain it, and fet the Liquor on the Fire, putting in two Blades of Mace, put in two Gills of Malaga, and Half a Pound of Currants, wafh'd and pick'd , and when they are plump'd, beat up the Yolks of two Eggs, and mix them with a little of the cold Broth, and thicken it over a flow Fire, keeping it ftirring all the while one Way : Seafon it with Salt, Sugar, Nutmeg, boil in it the Rhind of a Lemon, and juft before you difh it put in it the Juice of a Lemon.

Broth of Roots.

BOIL three Pounds of good white Peafe ; when they are very tender, bruife them to a Mafh, put them into a Pot that holds fix Chopins of Water, put it on the Fire for an Hour, ftrain it off and rub the Peafe thro' a Sieve ; then put it in a Pan with a Bunch of fweet Herbs,

Herbs, a shred Carot, six Onions, Parsley Roots, Sorrel, Chervil, Lettice, Endive and Sellery, a Handful of each: Season it with Salt, Pepper, Cloves, and *Jamaica* Pepper; boil it very well, it will be very good to put in any Herb Soup, or for a Soup with toasted Bread in it.

To make Cake-soup.

TAKE a Hough of Beef, a Knuckle of Veal, strip off the Skin and Fat, then take all the muscular and fleshy Parts from the Bones, boil the Flesh gently in three *Scots* Pints of Water, for so long a Time till the Liquor will make strong Jelly; try it if it is very strong before you strain it, by putting some to cool; strain it through a Sieve and let it settle, then let it be put in white Stone Cups, as clear as you can from the Settling, and set them in a Pan of cold Water, and put them on a slow Fire, and let the Water boil gently, till the Jelly is as thick as Glue; take care the Water does not go into the Cups, then let them stand to cool, and then turn out the Glue upon a Piece of Flannel, keep them turned every eight Hours on a dry Place of the Flannel till they are quite dry, then paper them in white Papers, and hang them up in a dry Place, there must be but one in every Paper: When you are going to make Use of them, boil an *English* Quart of Water, and pour it on them, keeping it stirring all the Time till it dissolves, it will make good Soup, season it to your Taste with Pepper, and put no Seasoning in the Glue; you may carry it in your Pocket, it will be good for Gravy or Sauce.

A Pottage of Goose Giblets.

SCALD and wash them clean, and cut them in Pieces, season them with Pepper, Salt, Onions, and a Bunch of sweet Herbs, boil them in good Broth till they are very tender, with some Crusts of
Bread

Bread in it; you may put green Peafe and fliced Lettices in it, take out the Herbs before you dish them.

A Muffel Soup.

GET a Pint of Muffels, fcald them and wash
them clean, put them in a Pan with three Mutchkins of ftrong Broth, and a Mutchkin of their own
Liquor, a Bunch of fweet Herbs, an Onion fluffed
with Cloves, Pepper, Mace and Salt, put in Crumbs of
Bread to thicken it, you may put a Gill of white Wine
in it; boil it till it is fmooth, you may fqueeze in it a
little Lemon Juice; fo ferve it up hot.

A Peafe Soup with Herbs in it.

BOIL two Pounds of Peafe in fix Chopins of Water till they are very foft, pour off fome of the Liquor,
and rub the Peafe thro' a Sieve, ftill putting in fome of
the Liquor to make them go through; then boil a
Pound of Butter, and when it breaks in the Middle, put
in an Onion and a little Mint cut fmall, Spinage, Sorrel, and Sellery cut grofly, let them boil a while, ftirring them often; then with one Hand fhake in fome
Flour, while with the other you pour in the thin Liquor; then ftir all together, feafon it with Pepper,
Mace and Salt, boil it for an Hour longer, then dish it:
You may put in a little fweet Cream if you pleafe.

To make Peafe Póttage.

TAKE two Quarts of Peafe, put them into three
Quarts of Water, feafon it pretty high with Pepper and
Salt, boil them till they are enough, mix a Spoonful
of Flour with Water, and put in a little Mint, a Leek,
two Handfuls of Spinage, all cut fmall, put in Half
a Pound of Butter, boil it and dish it.

A Turnip Soup.

PARE and cut in Dice twelve Turnips, which will
make a Dish full, fry them in clarified Butter a light
C   brown,

brown, put them in two Chopins of good Gravy and
the Crufts of fine Bread, let them drain from the Fat,
boil them till tender : You may put a Fowl in the
Middle.

A Hare Soup.

CUT your Hare in Quarters, and the reft in fmall
Pieces, put it in a Stew-pot with a Crag or Knuckle of
Veal, put in a Gallon of Water, a Bunch of fweet
Herbs, let it ftew till the Gravy is very good, fry a
little of the Veal and put in it to make it brown, put
in Bread to thicken the Soup, or you may put in Rice,
but boil it firft a little, or fine Barley; a Quarter of a
Pound of either will do; feafon it with Pepper, Salt,
and Mace, with an Onion ftuffed with Cloves; take
out the Herbs, Veal and Onion, before you dish it.

CHAP. II.

Of dreffing all Kinds of FISH, *and their Sauces.*

To ftew Carp or Tench.

WHEN they are catch'd put them in a Tub of
Water, kill them and fave all their Blood,
fcrape them, falt them well to take off the Slime, then
wafh and dry them very well in a Cloth: If they are
fmall, fry them firft, ftew them in a Mutchkin of Claret, and the fame of Gravy, a Piece of Butter work'd
in Flour, Pepper, Cloves, Salt and Mace, a whole
Onion, a Bunch of fweet Herbs, and an Anchovy, if
you have them; put Truffles, Morels, and Oifters in it
boil the Truffles, and Morels, fcald and pick the Oifters: Let your Sauce be boil'd, then put in you
Fifh and ftew them a good while, but don't let them
break

break: If the Sauce wants it, put in Ketchup; the large ones put in without frying, and ftew them on a very flow Fire, there muft be more Claret and Gravy in thefe than the fried ones; brown the Butter and Flour that you put in them that are not fried.

To drefs a Cod's Head.

IF you boil it, let your Water be boiling, put in it a Handful of Salt, a little Vinegar, and then put in your Fifh, be fure the Water covers it; if large, it will take an Hour to boil it, if fmall, Half an Hour; the fame Time bakes it, if the Oven is very hot: If baked, put Butter over and under it, the Sauce muft be either Oifters, Shrimps or Lobfters. Garnifh the Difh with Parfley, Horfe-radifh, and Forc'd meat Balls, and fliced Lemon.

To make Oifter, Lobfter or Shrimp Sauce.

PICK your Oifters clean and fcald them, ftrain their own Liquor and put it on them, then put Gravy if you have it, or a little Water in it, put in it a good Piece of Butter worked in Flour, a whole Onion, the Rind of a Lemon, Pepper, Salt, Nutmeg, and the Juice of Half a Lemon, you may put in Ketchup if you have it. The Lobfters muft be cut in Pieces, and white Wine in it.

To roaft or bake a Salmon.

SCORE it on the Back, feafon it with Salt, Pepper, Mace and Nutmeg; put grated Bread, the Grate of a Lemon, Parfley, Thyme, Salt and Butter in every Score, and in the Belly; put it in a clofs cover'd Pan in the Oven, with fome Butter on the Top and Bottom. You may give it either Oifter or Lobfter Sauce, or plain Butter.

To pickle Salmon.

TAKE a whole Salmon, and fcrape it clean, don't wafh it, cut it in round Pieces two Inches thick, ftrew
Salt

Salt on it to purge out the Blood. Make a ftrong Pickle of Salt and Water, whole Pepper, Mace and Cloves, with a Mutchkin of Vinegar and fix Bay Leaves; when it boils put in the Salmon, and let it boil a Quarter of an Hour; then take it out, and fet the Pickle to cool, fkim all the Greafe off it, then put in your Salmon. You may do large Trouts or Pikes the fame Way; if your Salmon is very thick, it will take more boiling.

A Turbot or any flat Fifh in Jelly.

WHEN your Fifh is well clean'd, let it lye in Salt two Hours, then wafh it and boil as much Water as will cover it, put in your Water Two pence Worth of Ifinglafs, Salt, Cloves, Mace and Pepper, and a Gill of Sherry, and one of Vinegar, put in your Fifh when the Liquor boils, and when you think it is enough, take it out and put on the Liquor again, and let it boil till it jellies, then beat the Whites of three Eggs and put in it, and give it four or five Boils more, then run it thro' a Jelly Bag, put your Fifh on the Difh, and when it is almoft cold, pour it on, Lemon Juice being better than Vinegar, and boil the Rind in it.

To broil Salmon.

BROIL fome Pieces of Salmon, feafoned with Pepper and Salt; for the Sauce put Butter, and Duft of Flour, a green Onion, an Anchovy, a little Ketchup, Oifter Liquor, a Glafs of white Wine, and the Juice of a Lemon, feafon it with Pepper, Salt, Nutmeg, and the Grate of a Lemon, difh your Salmon, and pour your Sauce about it; you may dip the Pieces of Salmon in melted Butter, and ftrew on them Crumbs of Bread and fweet Herbs fhred fmall, before you broil it, and the fame Sauce.

To farce Slices of Salmon.

CUT Slices of Salmon an Inch thick, take off the Skins, then mince fome of the Salmon, with fome

Eels,

Eels, Mushrooms, Chives and Parsley; season it with Pepper, Salt, Nutmeg, Cloves and Lemon-peel, pound them with a Piece of Butter; then put in it some Crumbs of Bread, and wet it with Eggs; dip the Salmon in Butter, and lay the Farce all over them; lay some Butter in a Dish, lay your Salmon in it, and cover it close; put it in the Oven; when baked, put it in the Dish, with either Oister, Lobster, or Cockle Sauce.

To hash Salmon.

HASH some Salmon in a Sauce-pan, dry it over the Fire till it grows white; then mince small some Mushrooms, Parsley, Shrimps and Oisters, and mince them all together; put some Butter in a Pan, with a little Flour; keep it stirring till it is brown; then put in the Salmon, give it a Turn or two on the Fire, season it with Salt and Pepper, and a little Juice of Lemon, put in a little Broth; serve it up hot.

To fry Salmon.

TAKE a Chine, or any other Part of Salmon, and cut it in Pieces, and fry them in clarified Butter or Beef Dripings, a little brown and crisp: For Sauce, put in the Sauce-pan some Claret, a Piece of Butter work'd in a little Flour, some Oister Liquor, the Juice of Lemon, and Nutmeg; put it on the Fire, and keep it stirring; dish the Fish, and pour it over them.

To bake a Turbot.

LAY some Butter in a Dish, the Size of the Turbot, and put Butter all over it; season it with Pepper, Salt, Cloves and Nutmeg, Crumbs of Bread, Lemon-peel, Chives, Parsley, a little Thyme, all shred small; flour it all over with it, bake it in the Oven a light brown, send it to the Table dry, with two Sauce-boats, one with Butter, the other with Oister Sauce.

To

To fry a Turbot.

SCORE your Turbot, flour it and fry it in clarified Butter, or good Beef Dripings; let it be boiling hot; then put it in and fry it a good brown, then drain it; make the Pan clean, put in it Claret or white Wine, Anchovy, Nutmeg, and an Onion, ſtuffed with Cloves and a little Salt; then put in your Fiſh, and let it boil a good while; then put in a Piece of Butter, work'd in a little Flour, and ſome Lemon peel, mix it well: Put your Fiſh in the Diſh, and pour the Sauce over it, but take out the Onion.

To ſouſe a Turbot.

BOIL it in Salt and Water, as much as will cover it, with a Mutchkin of Vinegar, Lemon-peel, Ginger, whole Pepper and Cloves; when boiled take it out, and when it and the Liquor is cold, put it in again with ſome Bay Leaves, and it will be fit to eat in two Days.

To ſtew a Turbot.

CUT it in Slices, and fry them; when they are half done, put them in a Stew-pan, with Claret, Lemon Juice, a ſliced Onion, Nutmeg, and a Bit of Butter; let the Fiſh ſtew till done; diſh it.

To cramp Cod the Dutch *Way.*

BOIL four Chopins of Water, and a Pound of Salt, ſkim it well; then put in the Slices of Cod, when it has boiled three Minutes it is done, then drain them well, and diſh them with raw Parſley about them; they muſt be cut very thin; they are eaten with Oil, Muſtard and Vinegar.

To ſtew Soals or any flat Fiſh.

SKIN your Soals, if they are large, on both Sides, and cut them in the Middle; if ſmall leave them whole, and ſkin them of the black Skin; the other

Fiſh

Fifh is not to be fkinned; have a Pan full of clarified Butter or Beef, or Beef Driping, boiling hot; flour your Fifh and put them in, fry them a light brown, then put them to drain all the Fat from them; brown a good Piece of Butter and Flour, and put to it fome Gravy, Oifter Liquor, a Bunch of fweet Herbs, an O-nion or two, Cloves, Mace, Pepper and Salt, half a Mutchkin of Claret, the Juice of a Lemon, and a chop-ped Anchovy; when they are well mix'd together put in your Fifh, and let them fimmer over a very flow Fire; if it is not thick enough, work a Bit of But-ter in Flour and put in it; half an Hour ftews them: You may put Truffles and Morels in them; take out the Herbs and Onions, garnifh your Difh with fliced Lemon.

To boil a Turbot or any flat Fifh.

PUT in your Fifh-kettle as much Water as will co-ver the Fifh, a Handful of Salt, two Gills of Vinegar, and a Stick of Horfe Radifh; put your Fifh in when the Water boils; an Hour boils a Turbot; the fmall Fifh lefs; you may give them Oifter, Lobfter, or Shrimp Sauce: Garnifh the Difh with Parfley, fliced Lemon, and Horfe Radifh; let your Fifh lie in Salt and Water ten or twelve Hours before you boil it: If you foufe your Fifh, you muft put in more Vinegar, Pepper, Cloves, Mace, Salt and Bay Leaves; take out your Fifh, then boil your Liquor better, put in whole Gin-ger and Lemon-peel, it will make your Liquor bet-ter; and when both is cold pour the Liquor on your Fifh: It is to be eaten cold with Oil, Vinegar and Muftard, or with fome of its own Liquor; you may put *French* white Wine in it with Vinegar. You may loufe Pike the fame Way.

To roaft or bake a Pike.

SCORE your Pike on the Back, rub it all over with melted Butter; make a Stuffing of Crumbs of Bread, Oifters,

Oisters, Lemon-peel, Parsley, Shalot, Thyme, sweet Marjoram and Anchovies, all shred small; put in as much Beef Sewet finely chopped as Bread; season it with Pepper, Salt, Cloves and Nutmeg; wet it with two Eggs, and lay a Lair of it in every Score, and put some in the Belly: Strew on the Fish Crumbs of Bread, Pepper, Salt, the Grate of a Lemon and Nutmeg, roll it up in the Caul of Veal or Lamb, or a very thick buttered Paper; tye it to a Spit and flame it well with Butter, or turn it round in a Dish, and put Butter about it. Put it in the Oven, and when done, drain all the Gravy from it, and make a Lobster or Oister Sauce for it; or you may take a little Gravy, a Piece of Butter work'd in Flour, an Onion stuffed with Cloves, a Gill of red or white Wine, the Gravy that comes out of the Fish, Oister Liquor and Ketchup. Garnish the Dish with fried Parsley, sliced Lemons, and shred Beet-roots and Pickles.

To make Oister Loaves.

GET five little *French* Loaves, cut a little round Bit out of the Top, and take out all the Crumbs, fry the Crusts, and boil them in clarified Butter · Take half a Hundred of large Oisters, scald and wash them very clean, crum the Pith of the Loaves, and put some of it in the Oisters, strain the Liquor to them, put grated Lemon and Nutmeg, a good Piece of Butter, a little Pepper, stir this in a Toss-pan on the Fire till it is very hot, then stir in a little white Wine, and a little Juice of Lemon, then fill your Loaves with it, let both be hot; put the Bit you cut off the Top on it again; you may make it without the Crumbs; thicken the Oisters with a little Cream and the Yolks of Eggs.

To dress a Pike with Oisters.

SCALE and gut it, wash it clean, cut it in Pieces, and put them in a Stew pan with a Gill of white Wine, a Half Mutchkin of Water, half a Gill of Vinegar, Parsley, Chives, Mushrooms if you have them, and
Truffles,

Truffles, Morels, and blanch'd Oisters, with their own Liquor, a Piece of Butter work'd in Flour, Pepper, Salt, Mace and Nutmeg; boil them all together, with a Bunch of sweet Herbs, and an Onion and Parsley must be shred.

To souse a Pike.

PUT the Pike into as much Water as will cover it, with Bay Leaves, Pepper, Cloves, Mace and Salt: Let it boil till it is tender, that a Straw may run thro' it; then take it up and put in the Liquor, white Wine and Vinegar: When your Liquor is cold put in your Fish. When it goes to the Table, garnish it with pickled Barberries, Lemon and Parsley; put some of its own Liquor about it.

To boil a Pike.

THRUST the Tail of the Pike in its Mouth, boil as much Water as will cover it, put in it a Gill of Vinegar, the Juice and Rind of a Lemon, a Piece of Horse-radish, put a Stuffing of forc'd Meat, made of Fish in the Belly; and when the Water boils, put in your Fish, and boil it with a quick Fire: For the Sauce, take a little of the Liquor it is boil'd in, an Onion stuffed with Cloves, the Liver minc'd, a Bunch of sweet Herbs, Pepper, Mace and Salt, put in Oisters or Cockles blanched, and pour on Liquor, a good Piece of Butter worked in Flour, a little white Wine and Ketchup; garnish it with Pickles and sliced Lemon.

To fry a Pike.

CUT it in Slices, put in it Verjuice, Salt, Pepper, Lemon juice, Chives, and Bay Leaves; let it lye Half an Hour, then dip them in a Batter and fry them, dish them garnish'd with slic'd Lemons and Parsley: Make your Sauce of brown'd Butter and Flour, Oister Liquor, Mushroom Liquor, Gravy of Fish or Flesh, Pepper, Salt and Mace, a little white Wine and Lemon Juice.

D

To bake Plaice or any flat Fifh.

CUT off the Heads; Tails and Fins; feafon them with Salt, Pepper, Nutmeg and Cloves, Parfley, fweet Herbs, Lemon-peel, Anchovies and Shalots; put Butter under and over them; ftrew on them Crumbs of Bread, bake them a fine Brown, cut all the Ingredients fmall, you may put in either Oifters, Cockles, or Shrimps, a Gill of white Wine, and the Juice of a Lemon. If the Difh is a handfome Difh you bake them in, you may fend them to Table in it, if not, take Care in taking them out; you may fend them as they are baked, with either plain Fifh Sauce, or Lobfter, or Shrimp.

To flew Soals.

PUT your Soals in a Stew-pan, with two Gills of white Wine, whole Pepper, Mace, Lemon peel and Salt; when they are half-ftewed, put in a little Butter work'd in Flour, ftir it till it is melted, then put in fome Oifters and their own Liquor, keep them often fhaking till the Fifh is enough. Squeeze in a little Juice of Lemons: Garnifh the Difh with Lemon and fried Toafts of Bread.

To boil Mullets, or flew them.

BOIL your Water and Salt, juft as much as will cover them; then put in your Fifh, with Vinegar and Horfe-radifh; take them up and let them drain, boil fome of their own Liquor, a Bunch of fweet Herbs, Onions, Pepper, Salt, Lemon-peel and Nutmeg, Ketchup, white Wine and Lemon Juice, thicken it with Butter and Flour, fo ferve them up, garnifhed with red Cabbage, fcraped Horfe radifh and fliced Lemon.

To pickle Smelts.

YOUR Fifh being wafhed and gutted, dry them in a Cloth; lay them in Rows, and put between every Row, Pepper, Nutmeg, Cloves, Mace and Salt, with the Powder of Cochineal, Salt-petre and Peter-falt, co

vel

ver them with Bay Leaves, then boil as much Vinegar as will cover them, and when cold pour it on them.

To roſt a Cod's Head.

SCORE it with a Knife, and ſtrew a little Salt on it, and lay it in a Stew-pan before the Fire, with ſomething behind it, throw away the Water that runs out of it the firſt half Hour; then rub it over with a little Butter, and ſtrew on it Nutmeg, Cloves, Mace and Salt, turn it often and baſte it with Butter If it is a very large Head, it will take four Hours roſting, take all the Gravy that runs out of it, and put more Gravy to it, and a Glaſs of white Wine, three Shalots, a little Horſe radiſh, Pepper, Cloves, Mace, Salt and Nutmeg, a good Lump of Butter work'd in Flour, the Liver of the Fiſh boiled, and chopped with Anchovies very ſmall, ſome Oiſters and Shrimps; thicken it with the Yolks of two Eggs, juſt as you're going to put it in the Sauce boat. Lay your Cod's Head on the Diſh, and put ſmall fried Fiſh and forc'd meat Balls, Slices of Lemons, Horſe-radiſh and Pickles over it, and ſend it up very hot.

To ſtew Cod.

CUT the Cod in thin Slices, lay it in a Diſh with a Mutchkin of Gravy, and two Gills of white Wine, ſome Oiſters and their Liquor, ſeaſon it with Pepper, Salt and Nutmeg, and let it ſtew till it is almoſt enough, then thicken it with a Piece of Butter roll'd in Flour, let it ſtew a little longer: Put in the Juice of a Piece of Lemon; ſerve it up very hot.

To broil a Cod

CUT the Cod in middling Pieces about an Inch thick, flour it well, and put it on the Gridiron over a flow Fire: The Sauce is a little Gravy, a Glaſs of white Wine, an Anchovy, Pepper, Salt, an Onion ſtuffed with Cloves, a Spoonful of Walnut Liquor; boil the Liver, chop it ſmall, and a Piece of Butter

rolled

rolled in Flour in the Sauce ; you may put in Oisters, Shrimps or Mushrooms , see that your Fish is well broil'd : Dish it and put Parsley about it.   Send your Sauce in a Boat.

To dress a Cod's Tail.

LOOSE the Skin that it may fall from the Flesh ; take the Fillets out, and make it with more Fish in Forc'd-meat, and fill up the void Spaces , then put the Skin upon the Tail again, rub it with Butter, and strew on it Crumbs of Bread, Pepper, Salt, and Lemon-peel, sweet Herbs shred small : Then put it in the Oven, and bake it a light brown.   You may make a Ragoo for it, or give it any Fish Sauce you please.

To stew Carps à la Royale.

WHEN they are very clean, put them in Claret, Salt, Pepper, Lemon-peel, an Onion stuffed with Cloves, Horse-radish and a little Vinegar , cover them closs, and let them stew gently on a slow Fire for three Quarters of an Hour , then beat some Butter, some of the Liquor that the Fish is stewed in, with two Anchovies chopped small, and some Oisters.   Dish your Carps on Sippets, and pour the Sauce over them.

To boil Carps.

SAVE the Blood. then boil them in a good relished Liquor for half an Hour , make the Sauce of the Blood, Claret and good Gravy, two Anchovies, two Shalots, whole Pepper, Cloves and Mace.   Let all stew together ; thicken it with Butter rolled in Flour, grate Nutmeg in it, and a little Lemon Juice , salt it to your Taste ; drain your Fish well : Dish them and pour the Sauce boiling hot over them.

To dress Eels with white Sauce.

SKIN and cut them in Pieces, blanch them, then dry them in a Napkin ; toss them up in Butter, with
Salt,

Salt, Pepper, Cloves, Lemon-peel, and a Glaſs of white Wine: Toſs up likeways ſome Artichoke Bottoms, Muſhrooms and Aſparagus, with Butter and ſavoury Herbs: Thicken the Sauce with the Yolks of Eggs; ſo ſerve them: Put Slices of Lemon and a little Juice in it.

To dreſs Eels with brown Sauce.

CUT your Eels in Pieces, toſs them up in clarified Butter and Flour; then put to them a little Fiſh Broth, Chives and Parſley ſhred ſmall, ſome Muſhrooms and Capers, a Bunch of ſweet Herbs, an Onion ſtuffed with Cloves, Pepper and Salt. When well boiled, put in a Glaſs of white Wine, and the Squeeze of a Lemon, and the Yolk of an Egg with Butter. So ſerve it up hot.

To fry Eels.

SKIN them, bone them, and cut them in Pieces, and lay them in Vinegar, Salt, Pepper, Bay Leaves, ſliced Onions, for two Hours; then drudge them with Flour, and fry them in clarified Butter. Serve them up dry with fried Parſley.

To dreſs Eels à la Daube.

MINCE the Fleſh of Eels, ſeaſon it with Salt, Pepper, Cloves and Nutmeg; cut the Fleſh of another Eel into Lardoons; then lay one Lair of them on the Skin, and another of the minced Fleſh, continuing ſo to do, till you have made it into the Shape of a Brick of Bread; put the Skin about it, and wrap it up in a Cloth, and ſtew it in half Water and half red Wine; ſeaſon it with Pepper, Salt, Cloves and Bay Leaf; let it cool in its own Liquor, and when you are going to ſend it to Table, cut it in Slices.

To roaſt a large Eel.

WASH it in Salt and Water, cut off the Head, and flea off the Skin a little below the Vent; gut it, wipe it clean with a Cloth, and give it three or four Scores with a Knife; then ſhread ſome Parſley, Thyme, and ſweet Marjoram, with an Anchovy, and ſome ſcalded Oiſters, mix them with Salt and Butter, and put them in the Belly of the Eel, and in the Scores; then draw the Skin over the Eel again, tye the Skin with a Pack-thread, to keep in the Moiſture; faſten it to a Spit, and roaſt it leiſurely, baſte it with Water and Salt till the Skin breaks, then baſte it with Butter; make your Sauce of beaten Butter and white Wine, with three or four Anchovies chopped in it.

To bake Tench.

WHEN they are well cleaned, lay them in a Pan with Gravy, white Wine, and ſome Muſhrooms, An-chovies, and three or four Shalots, ſome Pepper, Cloves, Mace, Salt and Lemon peel, with a Bunch of ſweet Herbs; lay ſome Butter all over the Fiſh, then cover them very cloſs, and bake them an Hour; then pour off the Liquor, and ſtrain it, only preſerving the Muſh-rooms; then add to it a Spoonful of Lemon Juice, and thicken your Sauce with the Yolks of three Eggs, mix it by Degrees with the Sauce, lay your Fiſh in a hot Diſh, and pour the Sauce over them.

To roaſt Tench.

HAVING cleaned it well from the Slime, make a Hole as near the Gills as you can, ſtuff the Belly as full of ſweet Herbs as you can, then tye it to the Spit, and roaſt it; mix Butter with Vinegar and Salt, and baſte it often; give it what Fiſh Sauce you pleaſe.

To fry Tench.

SLIT them down the Back, drudge them with Flour and Salt, then fry them, make the Sauce of Gravy,

Muſh-

Mushrooms, Artichoke Bottoms, Truffles, Anchovies and Capers, all chopped small, and well stewed; the Juice of a Lemon, and some Fish Cullis, or a Piece of Butter worked in Flour; boil it very well, send your Fish with Parsley on it, the Sauce in a Bowl.

To crimp Scate.

CUT the Fish the cross Way into ten Pieces, Inch broad, ten long, more or less, according to the Size of the Fish, then boil it quick in Salt and Water; put it dry on a Dish, and strew on it green Parsley; if it is to be eaten hot, put in one Cup Butter and Mustard, and in another Butter and Anchovy; send Oil and Vinegar to Table with it.

Flounders with Sorrel.

CUT three Scores on one Side of them, and lay them in a Pan with as much Water as will cover them, with a little Vinegar and Salt, boil them quick; then boil four Handfuls of Sorrel picked, and chop it very small; put it over the Fish, and pour half a Pound of melted Butter over it, drain the Fish very well.

To boil Flounders or Plaice.

PUT Salt, whole Pepper, white Wine, Vinegar, and a Bunch of sweet Herbs into your Water; let it boil apace before you put in your Fish; let them boil till they swim, then take them up and drain them; take a little of the Liquor, put in it some Butter work'd in Flour, two Anchovies and some Capers; beat it up thick on the Fire, then pour it in a Sauce Boat, put Parsley and sliced Lemon on the Fish.

To broil Flounders or Plaice.

SPLIT them, put Parsley and green Onions cut in a Stew-pan, with Pepper, Salt, and a Lump of Butter, put in your Plaice or Flounders, and turn them two or three Times to make them get a Taste, with-

out

out putting them over the Fire; then ſtrew them with Crumbs of Bread, and put them a broiling; when done, you may ſerve them up with any Sauce you pleaſe.

To ſtew Plaice or Flounders.

CUT them into, and place them in the Stew-pan, with as much Water as will cover them, put in a Blade of Mace, Salt, Lemon-peel, and a Spoonful of Lemon Juice, mix'd with Crumbs of Bread, Pepper, Nutmeg, Thyme, Parſley and Onion ſhred ſmall; then ſtew them on a ſlow Fire, lay the Fiſh in the Diſh, and pour it on them; or you may put them in the Pan with white Wine, Truffles, Muſhrooms, Parſley, Thyme, Chives, the Melts, and a little Butter and Flour, ſtir and turn them, but don't break them, put in the Yolks of two Eggs, well beaten; to fry them, only drudge them with Flour, and fry them brown, and put fried Parſley over them when brandered; the Sauce is melted Butter and Vinegar.

To dreſs Cabbolow.

BOIL it in boiling Water till it fleaks, put it on the Diſh, and ſtrew a good deal of hard Eggs, chopped fine over it, or you may leave the Fiſh in Heaps, and the chopped Eggs in Heaps; you may dreſs any ſalt Fiſh the ſame Way: If it is too dry, ſteep it before it is boiled, and ſend a Bowl of Butter and Muſtard to Table with it.

To pot Salmon, Trouts or Eels.

CUT off the Heads and Fins, ſcrape and wipe them very clean, cut them in middling Pieces, ſeaſon them very well with Pepper, Cloves, Mace and Salt, put them in a Can, and put a good deal of Butter about them, cover them with coarſe Dough, made of Meal; put them in a ſlow Oven: The Salmon will take an Hour baking, the reſt but half an Hour, when they come out of the Oven, take them out of the Can, and let them drain well from the Liquor, and let both cool, then take all the Butter off the Can, and clari-

fy

fy it with more Butter to cover your Fish, put them in small Pots, and pour the clarified Butter over it; you may send them to Table in the small Pots: If you find they don't come easy from the Bones, put them a while longer in the Oven.

To pot Lobsters or Scollops.

LET your Lobsters be as whole as you can, take them out of the Shell, and your Scollops quite whole, put them in different Pots, and the less the Pots are, the better; season them with Pepper, Salt, Cloves and Mace, put a good deal of Butter on them, put them in a slow Oven, and cover them; half an Hour bakes them, as they were boiled before; when cold, put clarified Butter over them.

To fricasey Oisters, Cockles or Mussels.

PICK them very clean, and strain a little of their own Liquor on them, with Crumbs of Bread, and a Piece of Butter work'd in Flour; season them with Pepper and Mace, a little Salt and Nutmeg, the Grate of a Lemon, a little white Wine, and the Juice of a Lemon, don't put too much Flour among the Butter.

To butter Crabs or Lobsters.

PICK all the Fish out of the Shell, put it in a Sauce-pan with Crumbs of Bread, Nutmeg, a very little white Wine, stir it about, and when hot, put it in the Shells, and some Crumbs of Bread on it, brown it before the Fire, and put the Juice of a Lemon in it, or a Lemon.

To make Caper Salmon.

TAKE out the Chine, salt it twelve Hours, then drain it well from the Salt and Blood, take an Ounce of Salt petre, and an Ounce of Peter-salt, and half a Pound of Bay Salt; rub it very well for six Days with this, then hang it up to dry by a slow Fire.

E

To keep Salmon in Pickle for a Year.

CUT off the Fins, and chine it, falt it for twenty Hours on a Board, boil a Pickle of Salt and Water, that will bear an Egg, as much as you think will cover the Salmon ; when your Pickle is almoft boiled, put in it an Ounce of Salt-petre, and an Ounce of Peter-falt, a Pound of Bay Salt, fkim it well, and when it is cold, pour it from the Bottom, then put your Salmon in it ; a Lime Can is beft to keep it in ; cut the Salmon in Pieces, as much as you think proper to boil at once.

To flew Haddocks or Whitings.

PUT them in the Pan, with a little Water, Pepper, Salt, Mace, chopped Parfley, Lemon-peel and Onion, a good Piece of Butter worked in Flour ; let them boil on a quick Fire. When you think they are enough, put in a little Wine, then take out tne Fifh, and thicken the Sauce with the Yolks of three Eggs well beaten, take Care it does not curdle : When you put Butter and Flour in any Thing, ftir it till it diffolves, fhread the Parfley.

To pot Herrings.

CUT off the Heads and Fins, put them in a Pan; feafon them with Pepper, Salt and Vinegar : If you put in a little Sherry in them, put the Juice of a Lemon inftead of Vinegar : Cover them clofs, and bake them in a flow Oven : They are to be eaten when cold. Eels may be done the fame Way.

To pickle Oifters, Scollops, Cockles or Muffels.

WASH and pick them clean in their own Liquor, then ftrain the Liquor, put them in it with whole Pepper, Cloves, Mace and Salt ; give them two or three Boils, then take them off, and eat them cold. A little of it is good in any Fifh Sauce.

To fcollop Oifters or Lobfters.

SCALD the Oifters, put them in the Scollop Shells, put a little Butter in the Bottom; feafon them with Nutmeg, the Grate of a Lemon, a very little Pepper, fome of their own Liquor, and a little white Wine: Put Crumbs of Bread over them; then put them in a flow Oven. Cut the Lobfter in Dice, and do it the fame Way. You may do them before the Fire on a Brander.

To ftew Eels.

CUT the Tails and Fins if large, fkin them, cut them three Inches long: Seafon them with Pepper, Salt and Cloves; put them in a Stew-pan, with a little Gravy or Water, a Bunch of fweet Herbs and two Onions: Cover them clofs, and let them ftew on a flow Fire. When the Fifh comes eafy from the Bone, they are done. Take out your Herbs, and put in Crumbs of Bread, and a little Butter worked in Flour, a Glafs of white Wine, and the Squeeze of a Lemon.

To make a Fricafey of Oifters.

PICK your Oifters very clean, put them on the Fire, and give them a Scald, fkim them and drain them clear from their own Liquor; ftrain the Liquor, put it in a Sauce pan with the Oifters, the Rind of a Lemon, an Onion ftuffed with Cloves, a Blade of Mace, a Piece of Butter worked in Flour; when the Rawnefs is off the Flour they are enough; put Sippets in the Afhet under them: Take out the Onion and Lemon-peel, and put a little white Wine, and the Juice of a Piece of Lemon in them, Pepper and Salt; thicken them with the Yolks of two Eggs.

To make Forc'd meat for Fifh.

CHOP a large Haddock very fmall, and put as much chopped Sewet as Fifh, and as much Bread, and a few chopped Oifters, feafon it with Pepper and Nutmeg,

meg, a little fhred Parfley, Onion, Salt and Lemon-peel; wet it with an Egg or two, fo roll it in fmall Balls, flour your Hands as you are rolling them; fry them in Butter a light brown, they will ferve any Sort of Fifh.

To fry Soals.

FLEA them, and drudge them with Flour, and get a Pan almoft full of clarified Butter, or good Dripings of Beef; when it is boiling hot, put in the Soals, and fry them a good Brown on both Sides; drain them very well from the Fat, put crifped Parfley and Slices of Orange over them. Or, you may give them a Sauce made thus: Take two Gills of Gravy, the fame of Claret, an Onion ftuffed with Cloves, Mace, and a little Salt or Anchovy Liquor, brown fome Butter and Flour, and ftir it in by Degrees, with chopped Mo-rels, and Forc'd meat Balls, you may put fried Oifters in it, and a little Oifter Liquor: Send it in a Sauce Boat.

A good Way to drefs Lobfters.

PARBOIL your Lobfters, break the Shells, pick out all the Meat, cut it fmall, take the Meat out of the Body, mix it fine with a Spoonful of white Wine, put it in the Stew-pan with the reft, cut the Tail in long Pieces, put in a Piece of Butter and a Gill of white Wine, fome Crumbs of Bread, a little Pepper, Salt, Nutmeg, and a Spoonful of Vinegar. Let it ftew a little, put in a Gill of Gravy. when hot, difh it.

Lobfters the Italian Way.

WHEN your Lobfters are boil'd, take the Meat out of the Tail and Claws, and cut it in Slices, put a little Butter in a Stew pan, Parfley, Mufhrooms and Truffles cut fmall, with a little Gravy, and a Glafs of white Wine; feafon it with Pepper, Salt. Nutmeg, fweet Herbs, and Rockambole: Let it ftew flowly, put the Meat of the Body and Juice of Lemon in it.

To dress Crabs.

TAKE the Meat out and cleanse it from the Skins, put it into a Stew pan, with two Gills of white Wine, some Crumbs of Bread, the Grate of a Lemon, Nutmeg, Pepper and Anchovy; put it on the Fire with a little Butter, stir it with the Yolk of an Egg, so dish it: You may put Claret instead of white Wine, if you please.

To make Water Sokey.

TAKE some of the smallest Flounders you can get, cut the Fins close, put them in a Stew-pan, and as much Water as will cover them; put Salt and a Bunch of Parsley, boil them till they rise to the Top: Send them to the Table with the Liquor about them; put Parsley and Butter in a Cup.

To stew Trouts.

PUT your Trouts in a Stew-pan, with two or three Gills of white Wine, and a Quarter of a Pound of Butter, Pepper, Salt and Mace, minc'd Parsley, Thyme, and green Onions: Let them all stew a Quarter of an Hour, then mince the Yolks of two Eggs and put them in. Dish them, and pour their own Liquor over them.

To spouse Trouts.

PUT all Sorts of Spice, and a Faggot of sweet Herbs, in as much Water and Vinegar as will cover the Fish, boil them in it: When they are enough, let them lye in the Pickle till you are for eating them.

To fry Lobsters.

TAKE a boiled Lobster, and take out the Meat as whole as you can, slice it the long Ways, flour it and fry it in clarified Butter; or you may make a Batter of Cream, Eggs, Flour and Salt, dip them in it and fry them: Then beat some Butter up thick, with grated Nutmeg, Claret and Orange Juice. Lay the Lobsters in the Dish, and pour the Sauce on it.

To

To stew Crabs.

BOIL them, take the Meat out of the Bodies, save the great Claws, mash the Meat that is in the Body, and mix it with Claret, Vinegar, Salt, Nutmeg, and a Piece of Butter: Put them in a Stew-pan with chopped hard Eggs, let them stew a good while, then put them in the Shells. Put them in the Dish with the Claws broiled round them.

To boil a Piece of Sturgeon.

TAKE a Rand of Sturgeon, put a Mutchkin of Vinegar, two Chopins of Water, some Slices of Lemon-peel, Horse radish, Bay Leaves, whole Pepper, Ginger, Cloves and Salt. The Liquor must boil before you put in the Fish: If it is to be eat hot, make the Sauce either of Oisters, Lobsters or Crabs; if it is to be kept in Pickle to be eaten cold, don't put in Vinegar, but put in a good deal of Salt, and all Sorts of Spices.

To roast a Piece of Sturgeon.

LAY your Sturgeon in Salt and Water six Hours, then spit it, and baste it well for a Quarter of an Hour; then drudge it with grated Bread, Nutmeg, Mace, Pepper, Salt, sweet Herbs, Lemon-peel cut small, continue drudging and basting till it is enough. Make the Sauce of Gravy, Oister Liquor, Lemon-peel, sweet Herbs, Onions, Ketchup, Pepper, Salt, Mace and some white Wine, strain it off, and put in as much Butter as will thicken it: You may put in either Oisters, Prawns, Lobsters or Crabs.

To fry Sturgeon.

TAKE a Piece of fresh Sturgeon, and cut it in Slices half an Inch thick, slash it and fry it in clarified Butter; then take it up and clean the Pan, and put in Claret, Lemon-peel, Nutmeg, Pepper, Salt and Anchovy. Let all stew a while, then put in a Piece of Butter roll'd in Flour and Shalot.

To fry Sperlings.

DRY them and rub them with an Egg, roll them in Crumbs of Bread, Lemon-peel, Parſley, Pepper, Salt, and fry them brown in clarified Butter. Send Parſley and Butter in a Cup.

To ſtew Sperlings.

PUT them in a Pan with a little Gravy, white Wine, the Yolks of three or four Eggs minc'd ſmall, a good Piece of Butter, an Onion ſtuffed with Cloves, a little Pepper and Salt. Let them ſtew till done; put the Squeeze of a Lemon in it. Send it up hot.

To boil Mackarel.

BOIL them in Salt and Water, with a little Fennel: The Sauce is the Fennel chopped ſmall, with beat Butter, or ſcalded Gooſeberries, with Butter and Sugar.

To pickle Mackarel.

CUT them in Pieces and ſeaſon them with Pepper, Salt, Mace and Cloves, rub them with it, and let them lye a while; then fry them in clarified Butter; then put them to drain; and when they are dry, put them in a Can, then boil Vinegar and Spiceries; and when it is cold, pour it on them.

To broil Mackarel.

WHEN they are well clean'd, draw them at the Gills, wipe them and ſtuff them with Crumbs of Bread, the Liver, Parſley, Pepper, Salt, Nutmeg grated, Lemon-peel, Shalot, and wet it with an Egg, then brander them, and when done pour over them beat Butter.

To fry Maids.

SKIN them and put them in Salt and Water, let them lye a while, then dry them with a Cloth; flour them, beat ſix Eggs, with a little Flour, Salt, Ginger, Nutmeg, Parſley ſhred ſmall, a little white Wine, beat

it

it up pretty thick; have a Pan with Beef Dripings, or clarified Butter boiling hot; dip your Maids in the Batter, and fry them brown. Let the Sauce be Butter, Vinegar, the Livers of the Fish, and Nutmeg beaten together; put fried Parsley over them, and the Sauce in a Boat.

To boil Gurnets.

STUFF the Bellies with Bread Forc'd meat, and boil them in Salt and Water; drain them well: The Sauce is beat Butter, Nutmeg, Lemon Juice, Shrimps, or Cockles, and a boiled Anchovy: When you broil them, you may give them the same Sauce, with a little Gravy in it.

To fry Whitings.

GUT them, and wipe them clean with a Cloth, and turn their Tails into their Mouths; make a Batter of Eggs, Flour and a little Salt; dip them in it, and strew on them Crumbs of Bread, then fry them a light brown. The Sauce is beat Butter and Anchovies, or Parsley and Butter.

To stew Scollops.

BOIL them very well in Salt and Water, take them out and stew them in a little of the Liquor, a little white Wine, Mace, Cloves, and a Piece of Butter rolled in Flour, a little Juice of Lemon and some Salt: You may do Cockles or Mussels the same Way; but scald them in their own Liquor.

To make a Collar of Fish.

TAKE a large Eel, skin it and pick off the Flesh, and beat it in a marble or wooden Mortar, season it with beaten Mace, Nutmeg, Pepper and Salt, sweet Herbs, Parsley, Lemon-peel and Shalots, all chopped small; beat all well together, with an equal Quantity of Crumbs of Bread; then take
any

any flat Fiſh that will roll, and lay it on the Dreſſer.
Take out all the Bones and Fins, and cover your Fiſh
with the Forc'd-meat; mix a Couple of raw Eggs
with it; then roll it up tight, and open the Skin of
the Eel, and bind the Collar with it, ſo that it may be
flat Top and Bottom. To ſtand well in the Diſh, butter an Earthen Can, and ſet it in it upright; flour it,
and put a Piece of Butter on the Top, and round the
Edges. Let it be well baked, but take Care it is not
broke, put two Gills of Water and a little Vinegar in
the Can, take another Eel cut in Pieces, and put it in
a Sauce-pan, with a Bunch of ſweet Herbs, Onion,
Truffles, Morels, and a few Muſhrooms, cover it cloſs,
ſeaſon it with Cloves, Mace, Pepper and Salt: When
well ſtewed, take out the Herbs and Onions, and put
in it a Bit of Butter work'd in Flour, a little Ketchup
and Lemon Juice. Make ſome of the Forc'd-meat in
little Balls, and fry them a light brown; when the Fiſh
is enough lay it in the Diſh, ſkim all the Fat off it, and
pour the Gravy to your Sauce, let it all boil together
till it is pretty thick; then pour it over the Roll, and
put in your Balls. Garniſh with Lemon and Pickles.

To ſtew a Pike.

LARD with the Fleſh of an Eel; then put it in a
Stew-pan, with ſome brown'd Butter and Flour, a little white Wine, Salt, Pepper, Nutmeg, an Onion ſtuffed with Cloves, Lemon-peel, and ſweet Herbs. Let
it ſtew on a gentle Fire, then put to it a Ragoo of
Muſhrooms, Oiſters, and the Liquor wherein they are
ſtewed. Diſh your Fiſh, pour over it the Ragoo, garniſh it with fried Oiſters, the Rands of Fiſh, Pickles,
and Slices of Lemon. When your Fiſh is ſtewing keep
it cloſe covered, put a little Verjuice in with the Fiſh.

F

CHAP.

CHAP. III.

To pot and make Hams, &c.

To pickle Tongues.

LET your Tongues be very well falted, and lye in it two or three Days, then make a Pickle for them: Put a Quarter of Salt petre, a Quarter of a Pound of Peter-falt, three Pounds of Bay Salt, and three of white Salt, in ten Chopins of Water; let it boil two Chopins away: See it be well skim'd; and when cold put it on your Tongues, but dry them firft in a Cloth. This Pickle will ferve either Pork, Geefe, or Sheeps Tongues. If you fee it grows muddy, boil it again, and put none of the Sediment in it. There muft be a Pound of coarfe brown Sugar in it.

To make Hams or Bacon.

SALT them on a Table, and lay a Weight on them for two or three Days, then to every Ham or Flitch of Bacon, take a Pound of white Salt, a Pound of Bay Salt, two Ounces of Salt-petre, and two of Peter-falt, a Quarter of a Pound of brown Sugar; mix them all together, and warm them pretty hot; lay your Hams in a Trough, and rub them very well, turn and rub them every Day for three Weeks; then hang them up to dry by a flow Fire: Wood, or Saw-duft, is the beft to dry them with.

To boil Hams.

IF they are dry foke them in cold Water, and put them in a Pot of cold Water with fweet Hay about them A large Ham will take three Hours to boil it, a fmall one but two, and a middling one two and a Half. If they are to be eaten hot, put Crumbs of Bread upon
them,

them; ſtuff the Ham with Cloves if you like it, and put it before the Fire.

To make Mutton Hams.

CUT the hind Quarter of very large fat Mutton like a Ham, then rub it all over with Bay Salt and brown Sugar; let it lye a Day, then put it in the Pickle, made thus: Take a Gallon of Pump Water, two Pounds of Bay Salt, two of white Salt, ſix Ounces of Salt-petre, and four of Peter-ſalt, one Pound of brown Sugar, one Ounce of Salt-prunella, put all in the Water, boil it well, and skim it. When cold, put in your Hams, let them lye in it a Fortnight; then hang them up and ſmoke them with Dale-duſt or Shavings; they muſt be dry before you make Uſe of them. You may pickle Bacon Hams the ſame Way, or any Sort of Tongues. When you hang up your Mutton Hams, boil the Pickle and skim it, and when cold you may put in Tongues, but ſalt them firſt for three or four Days.

Another Way to make Mutton Hams.

CUT the Mutton Ham-ways, take an Ounce of Salt-petre, a Pound of Salt, a Pound of coarſe Sugar, two Penny-worth of Cochineal, mix them, and rub the Ham very well, lay it with the Skin Side down, and rub it every Day for ſixteen Days, then hang it up to dry. It eats beſt in broil'd Raſhers.

To make Veal Hams.

CUT a Leg of Veal like a Ham; take a Pound of white Salt, a Pound of Bay Salt, two Ounces of Salt-petre, mix them and rub the Ham with it, lay it with the Skin Side down for a Fortnight, rubbing it every Day with the Pickle; hang it up, it will be dry in ſixteen Days. You may boil or roaſt it.

To make Beef Hams.

TAKE a fmall Leg of Beef, cut it Ham-fafhion;
an Ounce of Peter-falt and four Ounces of Bay Salt, a
Pound of white Salt, a Pound of coarfe Sugar; mix
them, and rub the Ham; lay it and all Hams in a Veffel at full Length that will hold the Brine; turn and
rub it every Day for a Month; then hang it to dry, but
not in too hot a Place.

To roaft an Ox or Sheep's Heart.

TAKE all the Blood out of it, and ftuff it with Forc'd-
meat, made thus: Take a Quarter of a Pound of Beef
Sewet, mince it fmall, two Handfuls of Crumbs of
Bread, Pepper, Salt and Nutmeg, Lemon-peel, Parfley,
Thyme, fweet Marjoram and Shalots, all fhred fmall:
Put in a chopped Anchovy, wet it with Eggs, and ftuff
the Heart with Cloves, or lard it if you pleafe; roll it
in buttered Papers, and roaft it well; it takes a good
deal of roafting, roll fome of the Stuffing in fmall
Bowls, fry them, and put them in the Dift with the
Heart, take off the Papers, and put Gravy under it.

To roaft a Haunch of Venifon.

RUB it over with Butter, and put on it a buttered
Paper, make a Pafte of Flour, an Egg and Water, and put
it on it, put the buttered Paper over it, tye it on with
Pack-thread, and put it to a good Fire, it takes three
Hours roafting if but fmall, more if large; take off
the Pafte and Paper, put Gravy under it, Claret Sauce
in a Boat, and Currant Jelly on a Saucer: If you boil a
Haunch of Venifon, let it be well falted for feven or
eight Days, then boil it in a large Pot of boiling Water,
fending it up with Colly-flowers, Savoys or Cabbage.

To roaft a Shoulder, or any Joint of Venifon.

LARD it with Bacon, feafon it with Pepper, Salt,
Nutmeg and Cloves, lay it four Hours in Steep of
white Wine, Lemon Juice and fweet Herbs, then fpit
it,

it, roaſt it at a gentle Fire, baſte it with its own Pickle; when roaſted, take what drips from it, and put to it Gravy, and a little Butter work'd in Flour, and Anchovy and Ketchup; boil it and pour it under the Veniſon, ſo ſerve it up.

To ſtew Veniſon that has been roaſted or baked.

GET a little Gravy, ſome brown'd Butter and Flour, a Gill of Claret, a Bunch of ſweet Herbs, ſome Shalots, Ketchup and an Anchovy, ſeaſon it with Pepper and Salt, boil it till it is ſmooth, then cut the Veniſon in thin Slices, and give it but one Scald; take out the Herbs, and ſqueeze in it the Juice of a Lemon, ſo ſerve it up hot.

To ſouſe Veniſon.

BOIL it in Water, Beer and Vinegar, ſkim it; then put in Thyme, Savoury and Bay Leaves, ſeaſon it with Pepper, Salt and Nutmeg.

To ſtew Veniſon.

CUT it in Slices, put it in a Stew-pan with Claret, Sugar, grated Bread, three or four Cloves, and a little Vinegar; let it ſtew for ſome Time, grate in Nutmeg, and ſerve it up; Veniſon may be haricot after the ſame Manner as Mutton is.

Veniſon in Blood.

THE Shoulder, Neck or Breaſt muſt be boned, and laid in Blood, ſeaſon it with Pepper, Salt, Winter Savoury, ſweet Marjoram and Thyme, all ſhred ſmall, with a little Beef Sewet chopped ſmall, and ſtirred on the Fire to be thick; then roll up the Veniſon with the ſet Blood and Herbs, and roaſt or ſtove it gently in good Broth or Gravy, Claret and Shalots; ſo ſerve it up hot.

To drefs Venifon à la Royale in Blood.

SPIT your Venifon, lay it down to the Fire till it is half roafted, then take it off and ftew it; make for it a Ragoo of Cucumbers, Sweet-breads and Afparagus.

To recover Venifon when it flinks.

TAKE as much Water in a Tub as will cover it, and put in a good deal of Salt, and let it lye three or four Hours; then take it out, and let it ly as long as before, in hot Water and Salt, take it out, and feafon it with Pepper and Salt, but dry it firft; put fome frefh Sheeps Blood in the Difh with it; it muft be high feafoned; don't ufe the Bones of the Venifon for Gravy, but put good frefh Gravy in it, cover it with Pafte; it will eat beft cold.

Venifon in Avet.

CUT it into Pieces the Bignefs of your Hand, lard it with Bacon, feafon it with Pepper and Salt, put it in a Stew-pan with Broth, white Wine, a Bunch of Herbs and Lemon-peel, the whole being ftewed, thicken your Sauce with Butter and Flour, and put a little Vinegar in it: It is a firft Courfe Difh; ferve it up hot.

A Civet of Venifon.

BOIL the Breaft or Neck, cut it into Cutlets, and when it is almoft boiled, brown half a Pound of Butter, and a good Handful of Flour; then add half a Pound of Sugar, and as much Claret as will make it of a good Thicknefs, then put in the Venifon, and give it three or four Boils, fo ferve it up; put the Juice of Lemon in it.

To keep Venifon all the Year.

A Haunch of Venifon being parboiled, feafon it with two Nutmegs, a Spoonful of Pepper, and a good Quantity of Salt; put to it two Spoonfuls of Vinegar, make the Venifon full of Holes, and put in your Spice and
Vinegar,

Vinegar, then put the Venison in a Pot, with the fat Side down, and cover it with two Pounds of Butter; then cover the Pot with coarse Paste, and bake it; when baked, take off the Paste, and lay a Trencher with a Weight on it, to keep it down till it is cold, then take off the Trencher, and lay the Butter flat all over the Venison, then cover it with Paper, and tye it down; send it to Table turned up Side down in a Dish.

To boil a Haunch of Venison.

SALT it for a Week, then boil it in boiling Water for two Hours and a Half, if large: Send it up with either Colliflowers, white Cabbages or Savoys, and melted Butter; you may boil any Joint the same Way, but don't salt it so long, or boil it so much.

To broil Venison.

CUT your Venison into Slices about half an Inch thick; season them with Pepper, Salt, and Crumbs of Bread; broil them over a brisk Fire. Serve them up with Gravy.

To make Venison Sokey.

BOIL the Venison, and make a Paste of the Crumbs of brown Bread, some Sugar, Pepper, Salt, Nutmeg and Orange peel minc'd small, and as much white Wine as will wet it: Mix all with your Hand, and wrap the Venison in it; set it into the Oven for an Hour; then serve it up with the white Wine boiled up with Sugar.

To roast a Fillet of Veal.

MINCE Beef Sewet very small, an Anchovy, Lemon-peel, Thyme, Parsley, sweet Marjoram, and an Onion; season it with Salt, Pepper, Nutmeg and Mace, add grated Bread to it: Mix all together with two Eggs, make Holes in the Veal, and stuff it with the Forc'd-meat; put a buttered Paper over it, that the

Stuffing

Stuffing does not come out. Spit it and roaft it well;
the Sauce is beat Butter, Gravy and Lemon: Garnifh
it with fliced Lemon, and red Beet Roots pickled.

To roaft a Shoulder of Veal with farcing Herbs.

PARBOIL it a little, then mince fome Thyme,
Parfley, Winter Savoury and Shalot, very fmall, and
mince fweet Herbs, chop four hard Eggs, a little Pepper, Salt and Nutmeg; mix all this up with two raw
Eggs, and ftuff your Veal with it, but fave fome of it;
fpit your Veal, roaft it, put your Stuffing in the Dri
ping pan, and when the Meat is near roafted enough,
put to it two Gills of Vinegar and a little Sugar. So
ferve it up.

To ftew a Knuckle of Veal.

PUT it in the Stew-pot with two Chopins of Water, four Blades of Mace, a little whole Pepper, a Sprig
of Thyme, an Onion ftuffed with Gloves, a Cruft of
Bread, cover it clofe, make it boil, then let it fimmer
for two Hours; lay it in the Difh, and pour the Broth
over it, take out the Thyme and the Onion, or you
may make the Sauce better, by putting in a little Ketchup, Walnut Pickle, Truffles, Morels and Mufhrooms.

To broil a Shoulder of Veal.

HALF roaft it, then flice off the moft Part of it,
and fave the Gravy, put the fliced Meat in a Stew-pan,
with a little Broth and its own Gravy, a little grated Bread, Oifter Liquor, Vinegar, fliced Bacon, a
Pound of Saufages out of their Skins made in Balls, and
rolled in Yolks of Eggs, Mace, Nutmeg, Salt, Lemon-
peel, and an Onion ftuffed with Cloves. Let all ftew
half an Hour, then put in a Mutchkin of Oifters, and
fome fweet Herbs; then take the Bone of the Veal and
broil it, and difh it: Then put in the Liquor, a Piece
of Butter work'd in Flour: let it boil, then pour it o-
ver

ver your broil'd Meat. Garnifh with fried Oifters, Barberries, and fliced Lemon.

To roaft a Calf's Head.

GET a Calf's Head with the Skin on, and fcald it, and boil it an Hour; when cold lard it with Lemon-peel; fpit and roaft it; when enough, make a Sauce of Gravy, Ketchup, Oifters, white Wine, Lemon, Forc'd-meat Balls, fried Sweet-breads, Mufhrooms, Truffles and Morels, put in a Piece of Butter work'd in Flour; boil all together, and pour over the Head. You may do it fkinned, if you pleafe.

A Calf's Head Surprife.

YOU muft bone it and not fplit it, clean it well, and fill up the vacant Place with Forc'd-meat, and make it in the fame Form as before: You may put in the Middle a Ragoo, and cover it with Forc'd-meat. Rub it with Eggs, and ftrew over it Crumbs of Bread and fweet Herbs, Lemon-peel fhred fmall; feafon it with Pepper, Salt and Nutmeg; bake it, and put a fa-voury Sauce under it. Blanch the Tongue, and let it hang out of the Mouth.

To boil a Calf's Head.

BOIL and bone it, then have in Readinefs the Pa-late boil'd tender, Yolks of hard Eggs, Oifters fcalded, and Forc'd meat; feafon it with Pepper, Salt and Nut-meg: Stuff all in the Head, tie it in a Cloth, boil it three Hours, put Gravy under it, garnifh it with Ba-con.

Beef à la Daube.

GET a Buttock of Beef, lard it, and force it with Forc'd meat, then pafs it off brown, put in fome Broth and a Faggot of fweet Herbs, feafon it with Pepper, Salt, Cloves, Mace, ftove it four Hours very tender, and make a Ragoo of Morels, Truffles, Mufhrooms, Artichoke Bottoms, Sweet Breads and Palates, white

G

Wine

Wine and Lemon Juice. Garnifh with Petty-Patees and Pickles.

To make Efcarlot Beef.

TAKE a Brifket of Beef, half a Pound of coarfe Sugar, two Ounces of Bay Salt, one Ounce of Salt-petre, a Pound of common Salt: mix all together, and rub the Beef, put it in an Earthen Pan, and turn it every Day: Let it lie a Fortnight in the Pickle, then boil it with Savoys, or a Peafe Pudding. It eats very well cold.

Beef la Vinaigre.

GET a Slice of Beef three Inches thick, moft lean, from the Buttock, ftew it with a little Water, and a Gill of white Wine; feafon it with Pepper, Salt, Cloves, a Faggot of fweet Herbs, and a Bay Leaf: Let it boil till it is very tender, then fet it a cooling, and when cold ferve it up, with Slices of Lemon and a little Vinegar.

To roaft a Tongue and Udder.

BOIL the Tongue till it will blanch, put it in cold Water, it will blanch the better, then lard it with Fat of Bacon an Inch long, and ftuff the Udder with Cloves, then fpit and roaft them, bafte them with Butter. Serve them up with Gravy, but fend in a Boat Claret boiled thick as a Syrup, with Sugar and Currant Jelly, or a favoury Sauce.

Or Tongues à la mode.

BOIL and blanch and lard it, then brown it off, and ftove it one Hour in good Gravy and Broth, feafon it with Pepper, Salt, Cloves, and a Faggot of fweet Herbs, put in Morels, Truffles, Mufhrooms, Sweet breads, and Artichoke Bottoms; fkim off the Fat, and ferve them either hot or cold.

To collar Beef.

TAKE a broad Runner of Beef, bone it, rub it with white Salt and Salt-petre, turn it and rub it every

Day

Day for eight Days; then dry it in a Cloth, and season it with Pepper, Cloves, and *Jamaica* Pepper; roll it very hard, and put it in a Cloth, bind it with broad Netting, and put it in a Pot of boiling Water, let it boil three Hours, then take it up and hang it by one End, and when it is almost cold take it out of the Cloth: It is to be eaten cold, you may send it to Table, either whole or in Slices. You may collar a Flank the same Way, but take off the Skin.

To stew a Rump of Beef.

CUT off the large Bone, that it may lye flat in the Stew-pan, score the Inside, and season it with Pepper, Salt, Cloves and Mace; shred a little Thyme, Parsley, Winter Savoury, and sweet Marjoram; put Seasoning between every Score if you like it; lard it with Bacon, and a Slice of Bacon laid in every Score. Put it in your Stew-pot with a Pint of Water, a little Rockambole or Shalots; let it stew on a gentle Fire for two Hours, then turn it, and make a Ragoo of Palates and Eyes, Forc'd-meat Balls and Kernels, with some of the Liquor it is stewed in; thicken it with brown'd Butter and Flour: Put in your Ragoo a half Mutchkin of white Wine and the Juice of a Lemon, the Grate of a Nutmeg, and Mushrooms if you have them. You may make a Ragoo for it if you please the same Way, of Carots, Turnips, Artichoke Bottoms, Truffles, Morels, Mushrooms and Oisters: You may stew any Piece of Beef the same Way. Boil your Roots before you put them in your Ragoo.

To make Dutch Beef.

TAKE six Pound of a Buttock of Beef, without Bones, rub it all over with five Ounces of coarse Sugar, let it lye two Days, then wipe it, and take a Mutchkin of white Salt, two Ounces of Salt-petre, and three of Peter salt, dry all before the Fire, and rub it well into the Beef; then put it in a brown glazed Pan
that

that will hold the Beef, and turn it, and rub it every Day for three Weeks : Then put it in a Canvas Bag, and hang it up in any Place where it will dry gradually, turn it often that the Brine does not settle, When dry boil it, and you may either slice or scrape it when it goes to Table.

Beef Steaks with Oyster Sauce.

CUT your Steaks off any tender Part of the Beef, flat them with your chopping Knife, and put them on a hot clean Brander, on a clear quick Fire, turning them often, that the Gravy does not run out, have your Sauce ready, make it thus: Scald your Oisters, and wash them clean in their own Liquor, then strain the Liquor into a Sauce-pan, put to it a Piece of Butter work'd in Flour, two or three Shalots, pounded Pepper, Cloves and Nutmeg, salt it to your Taste, put a Glass of white Wine, and the Rind and Juice of a Lemon in it : So pour it on your Ashet of Steaks boiling hot. Garnish them with Pickles.

To make hung Beef.

TAKE a Surloin of fat Beef, salt it well with white and Bay Salt, Salt petre and brown Sugar, let it lye in it for a Fortnight, turning and rubbing it every two Days; then hang it to dry; it eats well either in Rashers, or with Fowls and Greens, but it must not be cut till it is thorough dry.

To boil a Rump of Beef the French Way.

BOIL it for half an Hour, take it up in a deep Dish, cut Gashes in the Side to let out the Gravy, then put Pepper and Salt in every Gash, then fill the Dish with Claret and some Blades of Mace, set it on a chaffing Dish of Coals, and cover it closs, and let it stew an Hour and a Half. Turn it often, take off all the Fat, put in a Handful of Capers, five Onions, and six hard Lettuces, slice them both, put in a Spoonful of Verjuice;

juice; boil all till the Meat is tender. So serve it up on Sippets.

To stew a Rump of Beef.

BOIL it till it is half enough; take it up and peel off the Skin; then take Pepper, Salt, Mace and Nutmeg, Parsley, sweet Marjoram, Savoury and Thyme shred, stuff them in large Holes thro' the Fat, and lay all the rest of the Seasoning over the Top, and lay it all over with Eggs to bind it; put the Gravy that comes out, with a Mutchkin of Claret and a Gill of Vinegar, in a deep Pan with the Liquor, you may fill it to the Top. Cover it, and bake it four Hours; then put it in a Dish, and pour the Liquor over it.

To grillard a Breast of Mutton.

HALF boil a Breast of Mutton, score it in Dice, then rub it over with an Egg; take Crumbs of Bread, Pepper, Salt, Thyme, sweet Marjoram, Chives and Parsley; mix all together, and lay it on it, then broil it gently, for Sauce take Butter, Gravy, Capers, Shalot and Cucumbers, all shred small; garnish it with pickled Onions, red Cabbage, and Kidney Beans.

To make Mutton Cutlets.

CUT a Neck of Mutton in single Bones, flat them with the Chopping-knife, season them with Pepper and Salt, rub them with Eggs, and lay all over them Forc'd-meat; make it thus: Chop a little of the lean Mutton, with twice as much Sewet, as much Crumbs of Bread as Mutton, Pepper, Salt, the Grate of a Lemon, Parsley, Thyme and Shalot; chop all very small, and mix them up; wet them with Eggs, roll your Cutlets, in buttered Papers, and broil them on a clear Fire: They will take a Quarter of an Hour: When done, take them out of the Papers; the Sauce must be Butter and Gravy, Lemon and Ketchup: You may do Veal the same Way, but it takes longer broiling; garnish them
with

with Pickles; if Veal, with Lemon, Mushrooms, and Beet Roots.

To roast a Collar of Mutton.

BONE a Breast of Mutton, and rub it with Eggs, lay all over it Forc'd-meat, made as above roll it up very tight, and bind it closs: You may tye it on a Spit, or do it in the Oven; make a Hash to put under it, cut your Mutton in thin Bits, brown a little Butter and Flour, put in a little Gravy, put a Bunch of sweet Herbs, the Rind of Lemon, and two Onions stuffed with Cloves, Pepper and Salt, boil it well, then put in your Hash with Mushrooms, Cucumbers, and Kidney Beans, mince it, but not small: Don't let your Mutton boil, but give it a Scald or two; it must be roasted before you cut it, put it on the Dish, and the Collar over it, take off the Binding, and throw out the Onions and Herbs: Put Lemon Juice in the Hash. Garnish with Pickles.

To roast a Leg of Mutton with Oisters.

TAKE some Crumbs of Bread, a little Beef Sewet, some hard Eggs, an Onion, three Anchovies, Thyme, and Winter Savoury, twelve Oisters, Lemon peel and Parsley, mince them small, season it with Pepper, Salt and Nutmeg; mix all these together, and wet them with raw Eggs, stuff the Mutton under the Skin in the thickest Place, and half roast it; cut off some of the Under-side of the fleshy End in little Bits, put them in a Sauce-pan, with a Mutchkin of Oisters and their Liquor, season them with Mace and Salt; put in a good Piece of Butter in Flour, and when the Mutton is done, dish it, and pour the Sauce round it.

A Shoulder of Mutton in Epigramme.

TAKE a Shoulder of Mutton, half roast it, and take off the Skin as neatly as you can, the Thickness of a Crown, leaving the Shank-bone to it; then cut

-the

the Meat in thin Slices, the Bignefs of a Shilling; put it into good Gravy with a Piece of Butter, fome grated Bread, Pepper, Salt and Nutmeg, an Onion, Anchovy, and Pickles fhred; rub the Skin over with an Egg, and ftrew it with Crumbs of Bread, Pepper, Salt, Chives and fweet Herbs, fhred fmall: brander it, but don't let the Hafh boil much · difh the Hafh, and put on it the broiled Bone and Skin; you muft not cut them a-funder.

Carbonaded Mutton.

CUT a Joint of Mutton in Steaks, and fry them; then ftew them in good Broth, with Crumbs of Bread, a Bunch of fweet Herbs, Mufhrooms, Salt, Pepper and an Onion ftuffed with Cloves, take out the Herbs and Onion before you fend it up.

To boil Sheeps Tongues with Oifters.

BOIL fix Sheeps Tongues in Water and Salt till they are tender, peel off the Skin, cut them in thin Slices, put them in a Stew Pan with a Chopin of Oifters, a little Claret, Cloves and Mace, fet them a ftewing, then put in fome Butter, and the Yolks of three Eggs well beaten, fhake them well; don't put in the Eggs till you are going to difh them. You muft not let the Eggs boil in them, but be fcalding hot.

To roaft a Calf's Head with Oifters.

CUT the Head as for boiling, take out the Brains and the Tongue, parboil them, blanch the Tongue, and mince them with a little Sage, Beef-fewet and Oifters, with Yolks of Eggs and Crumbs of Bread, Pepper, Salt, Nutmeg, grated Lemon-peel; parboil and dry the Head, fill the Skull with thefe Ingredients, then ftuff it with Oifters, and faften it to the Spit, as it roafts preferve the Gravy, put to it a Glafs of white Wine, Salt, Nutmeg, Lemon-peel and Shalot, a Piece of Butter work'd in Flour, fome Oifters, and

a

a little Lemon-juice, beat it up thick. When the Head is done, dish it, and pour the Sauce about it.

To dreſs Calves Feet.

BOIL them tender, ſlit them in the Middle, put them in a Stew-pan with a Gill of Gravy, a Piece of Butter, a little Onion, Parſley chopped ſmall, Pepper and Salt, a Spoonful of Vinegar, ſtew them all together, ſo diſh them. You may make them ſweet, and put Currants and white Wine in them; thicken them with the Yolks of two Eggs.

Cakes of Beef to be fried or brandered.

CHOP ſome of the tendereſt Part of the Beef very ſmall, and pound it as much as for Sauſages, mix Half the Quantity of Beef-ſewet with it, ſeaſon it with Pepper and Salt, you may put Onions and Parſley in them, wet them with an Egg, make them in Cakes, and fry them in their own Gravy, or brander them on Papers.

To force the Inſide of a Surloin of Beef.

LIFT up the Fat carefully, cut out the Meat to the Bone, and chop it ſmall; cut a Pound of Sewet fine, and as many Crumbs of Bread, a very little Parſley, Lemon-peel, and two Shalots; ſeaſon it with Pepper, Salt and Nutmeg, mix all together with a Glaſs of Claret and raw Eggs; then put it in the ſame Place, and skewer the Fat over it. Paper it, and don't take off the Paper before you diſh it. You may put Gravy or Claret to it. Spit the Meat before you put in the Forc'd-meat.

A Neat's Tongue the Poliſh *Way*.

BLANCH off the Skin and boil it, cut it in two, but not quite off; ſtick it with Slices of preſerved Lemon, and Bits of Cinnamon; then put a Bit of Sugar, a Glaſs of white Wine, and a little Gravy: Then let the Tongue ſtew a while, and diſh it with the Sauce about it.

To

To fry a Neat's Tongue.

BOIL and blanch it, then cut it in thin Slices, season it with Nutmeg, Cinnamon and Sugar, dip them in the Yolks of Eggs, put some Butter and a little Vinegar in a Pan, and when it is boiling hot, drop in the Tongue and Eggs by Spoonfuls; when they are done dish them. The Sauce is beat Butter, white Wine and Sugar.

To stew a Neat's Tongue whole.

PUT a raw fresh Tongue in a Stew-pan with good Broth, white Wine, Pepper, Salt, Cloves, Mace and Capers, with Slices of Carots and Turnips. Set this over a gentle Fire, and let them stew two Hours, then take up the Tongue and blanch it, and put some Marrow to it, and let it have a Boil or two, and dish it on Sippets, and pour all over it.

To bake Ox cheeks.

LET them lye in Water all Night, then bone them and stuff them with Cloves, season them with Pepper, Salt and Mace; put them in a Pan, one Cheek laid close upon the other: Put Bay Leaves on them and a Chopin of Claret, cover the Pan close and bake them well. When they are baked pour off the Fat, and mix it with melted Butter, and pour over the Cheeks. They are to be eaten cold with Mustard and Sugar, the Gravy is to be all poured from it before you put the Butter on.

To roast a Leg of Mutton with Cockles

STUFF it all over with Cockles and roast it. Put Gravy under it.

To pot beef.

TAKE a Buttock of Beef, and cut off some thin Slices, and strew on it a little Salt-petre, let it lye four days in it, turning it every Day; then put it in a Can with sweet Butter, or sweet Sewet shred small: Cover it with a coarse Paste made of Meal, and bake it in a hot Oven for three Hours; then take it out, and take all the Greafe and Gravy from it; when it is cold ftring it and pound it fine, then feafon it with Pepper, Salt, Cloves, and Nutmeg, then draw fome fweet Butter to Oil, and fkim it, and pour it from the Bottom; to every two Pound of your pounded Meat put a Pound of your oiled Butter, and work it up well together, put it in fmall white Patees, and, when cold, melt fome Butter, and pour it on them. You may pot Venifon the fame Way.

To make Beef Ollops.

CUT thin Slices of Beef where it is tender, and beat it well with your Rolling pin; then feafon it with Pepper, Salt, Cloves, Mace and fweet Herbs, and Lemon-peel very fine, feafon it with Spice as above. Lay a Lair of this all over your Ollops, and roll them up tight; put them in a Can with a little Butter, cover them clofe and bake them, when they are done, take them out in Slices, and put them on a Difh, pour on them fome of their own Gravy, with a little white Wine and the Juice of a Lemon: Don't make it four, you may thicken it with a little Butter and Flour, grate Nutmeg in it.

To make Veal Collops.

TAKE a hind Quarter of Veal, and cut the thick Part in very thin Slices, beat them with a Rolling pin, feafon them with pounded Mace, Cloves, Pepper, and the Grate of a Lemon, then fry them a light brown in fweet Butter, when they are fried, get fome good brown Gravy, and thicken it with a little Butter and Flour, boil it with an Anchovy, and a whole Onion, a little Ketchup, and the Juice of half a Lemon: when boil'd put in your Collops, and give them one Boil, if they are not feafon'd enough, put in more of that you feafon'd your Collops with, put Forc'd meat and an

Anchovy,

Anchovy, and a little Salt. You may put Mushrooms in them and Oisters, but scald them first.

To make Forc'd-meat Balls.

CHOP some of the tenderest Part of Veal or Mutton, very fine, with an equal Quantity of Beef or Mutton Sewet; season it with Pepper, Salt, Nutmeg, Cloves, and the Grate of a Lemon, and a little sweet Herbs, wet it with two Eggs, and work it together with your Hand, make it in small Balls, and fry it in sweet Butter: Flour your Hands when you roll them.

Another Sort of Forc'd meat Balls.

CRUMB a Penny Loaf, and add to it eight Ounces of Butter, or Beef Sewet, minc'd very fine, Lemon-peel, Parsley, and a Bit of Onion shred fine; season it with Pepper, Salt, Nutmeg, wet it with two Eggs, roll it in your Hands to a Paste, then make it in small Balls the Bigness of a Nutmeg, fry them in Butter.

Another Sort of Forc'd-meat Balls.

CHOP an equal Quantity of any tender Meat, with Beef or Mutton sewet, and the same Quantity of Crumbs of Bread, with Lemon peel, Parsley and Onion shred small; season it with Pepper, Salt, Nutmeg and Cloves. Wet it with Eggs, and work it up together, then roll it in small Balls. Fry them in Butter.

To make Veal Fricardos.

CUT a Neck of Veal in Chops, letting two Bones be together, put them in a Stew-pan with a little Water, Lemon-peel, Onions, Pepper, Salt, Mace and Anchovy, and a little sweet Herbs tied in a Bunch, let it stew on a slow Fire till the Head is boil'd; then take out your Herbs, Lemon-peel and Onions, and thicken it with Butter work'd in Flour, put a little white Wine and the Juice of a Lemon in it, and Mushrooms if you

have

have them, and some boil'd Artichoke Bottoms cut in Dice.

To force a Leg of Mutton or Lamb.

CUT all the Meat out, but don't break the Skin, to every Pound of Meat put Half a Pound of Beef or Mutton Sewet, chop them very fine, shread sweet Herbs, Lemon-peel and Shalots, mix them with it, season it with Pepper, Salt, Cloves and Nutmeg, wet it with two Eggs, mix all together, and fill the Skin, spit it, and roll about it a well buttered Paper: Tye it closs that the Stuffing does not come out, it will take a good while to roast it. Put Gravy in the Dish with it, and a Ragoo of Palates and Sweet-breads: Fry the Loin, and lay it round it.

To make a Mutton or Lamb Hash.

HALF roast either a Shoulder or Jiggit of Mutton or Lamb, cut it in thin Slices; save the Gravy; put it in your Pan with a little Butter work'd in Flour, some Pickles, Pepper, Salt, Ketchup, Onions, and the Rind of a Lemon cut small; if it is too thick, put in a little Water: Two or three Boils does it.

To make minc'd Collops.

TAKE any Part of the Beef that is tender, and mince it small, to every Pound of it put a Quarter of a Pound of Sewet minc'd very fine, put it in a Tofs-pan, with a little Gravy or Water, and some Onions shred small, season it with Pepper, Salt and Cloves: Let it stew on a slow Fire till it is tender, then work a very small Bit of Butter in Flour, and give it a Boil in it, so serve it up. You may put Pickles in it if you please.

To make Beef Collops.

CUT your Collops broad, and very thin, flat them with your Chopping Knife, flour them, and fry them a light brown: Make your Sauce of Gravy, a little Butter work'd in Flour, and a little Ketchup; season it

with

with Pepper, Salt, Mace and Onions: When boil'd
put in your Collops, and Pickles with them. You may
do either Lamb or Mutton the same Way. Don't
boil your Meat in the Sauce, but pour it over them:
You may brander them, and pour the same Sauce with
Oisters on them.

Entry of Sheeps Trotters forced.

SCALD the Trotters, and let them stew in a little
Water well seasoned; take them up when the Bones
will come out, stretch them on a Table, put Forc'd-
meat in them, and roll them up one by one; place
them in a Dish, and moisten them with a little Butter;
strew on them Crumbs of Bread, Pepper, Salt and
sweet Herbs; put them in the Oven; when brown,
dish them, and put a Ragoo Sauce on them.

Veal Olives.

TAKE ten or twelve thin Veal Collops, rub them
over with an Egg; then lay on them Forc'd-meat, and
roll them up, toast or bake them: When done, pour
over them a Ragoo of Sweet-breads. Garnish the
Dish with Oranges.

Another Way.

TAKE the Flesh of a Fillet of Veal, and half the
Quantity of Beef Sewet chopped very small, add to
it Mushrooms, Oisters, and two Anchovies, chop them
all small, season them with a little Thyme, sweet
Marjoram, Parsley, Lemon-peel, all shred small; Pepper, Salt, Nutmeg and Mace; then take the Veal Caul,
and lay it all over with the Forc'd meat: You may
roll it in two or three Collars; roast or bake it, when
done, cut it in Slices, and serve it up with strong Gravy.

To stuff a Rump or Round of Beef.

CHOP two Handfuls of Parsley very small, and one of Beef Sewet shred small; mix them and Pepper and Salt together, make Holes with a Knife in the Beef, and stuff them full of it: The Beef is to ly salt four Days before it is stuffed, boil it tender. You may eat it either hot or cold.

White Scots Collops.

CUT the Veal into thin Slices, beat them with the Rolling-pin: You may lard them if you please, season them with Pepper, Salt, Cloves, Mace, Lemon-peel and grated Bread, dipping them first in Eggs, stew the Knuckle well, with a Bunch of sweet Herbs, two Anchovies, Cloves, Mace, Pepper and Salt; strain it, and when you are going to send it up, thicken it with a Bit of Butter work'd in Flour; give it two or three Boils, then put into it the Yolks of three Eggs well beaten, a Glass of white Wine, and the Juice of a Lemon, and give it a good Heat on the Fire, but don't let it boil, stirring it all the while. Your Collops being fried, but not brown, lay them in the Dish, and pour your Sauce over them. Garnish it with Mushrooms and Oisters; don't make it too sour.

To stew a Knuckle of Veal.

LAY at the Bottom of your Pot four long wooden Skewers, wash the Veal, and lay it in the Pot with three Blades of Mace, some whole Pepper, a Sprig of Thyme, a small Onion, a Crust of Bread, and two Quarts of Water, cover it closs, and let it come to the Boil, then let it only simmer for two Hours, then take it up, and strain the Broth over it; put young Pease or Asparagus in it.

Lamb with Rice.

HALF roast a fore Quarter of Lamb, put a Pound of Rice into two Quarts of good Broth, three Blades,
of

of Mace, Salt and Nutmeg; let it ftew an Hour; take it off, and put in the Yolks of four Eggs, and a Pound of Butter; then put in the Lamb in Joints in a Difh, with the Rice over it, wafh it with Eggs, and bake it half an Hour: You may do Hens or Chickens the fame Way, but leave them whole.

To make a Calf's Head Hafh.

HALF boil your Head, and cut the one Half in thin Slices; put it in your Pan with Gravy, a Bunch of fweet Herbs, the Rind of a Lemon, a whole Onion, and an Anchovy; feafon it with Pepper, Salt, Mace and Nutmeg. When it is almoft boiled, thicken it with Butter work'd in Flour; put in a little fweet Cream: Score the other half, and ftrew on it Crumbs of Bread, fhred Parfley, Lemon-peel, Pepper, Salt and Nutmeg; put it in the Driping-pan to brown, bafte it with Butter; when done, put it in your Difh and before you pour your Hafh about it, put in a little white Wine, fome Lemon Juice and Mufhrooms, if you have them, and Oifters; you may make it brown without Cream.

To make a Lamb's Head Hafh.

BLANCH and clean your Head very well, half boil it, cut the Haricals in thin Slices, and take a little of the Water it is boiled in, and put your Hafh in it, with an Onion ftuffed with Cloves, the Rind of a Lemon, Pepper and Salt, a little Ketchup; thicken it with Butter work'd in Flour, take out the Brains, and mix them with Crumbs of Bread, grated Lemon-peel, Nutmeg, Pepper, Salt and an Egg, then put them in the Head again, and lay it in the Driping-pan till it is well roafted, then put it in your Difh, and pour your Hafh round it. Garnifh all your Hafhes with Lemon, and put a little of the Juice in them.

Another

Another Way to drefs a Lamb's Head.

HALF boil the Head, cut it through the Scull in.
to Halves, take out the Brains, mince the Haricals fmall,
and the Brains amongft them, put them in a Stew-pan
with a little Gravy, or fome of the Water that they
were boiled in, with a little Butter work'd in Flour,
the Grate of a Lemon, Onion, and Parfley minc'd fmall,
a little Ketchup, the Squeeze of a Lemon, Pepper, Salt,
and Nutmeg; boil all together, put the Head in a Driping-pan, rub it over with an Egg, and throw on it
Crumbs of Bread, fweet Herbs fhred fmall, Pepper,
Salt and Nutmeg; bafte it with Butter. When it is
done enough, put it on the Difh with the Hafh about
it, fry the Liver in thin Slices, and put it about your
Difh.

To ftew a Lamb's Head.

PUT the Lamb's Head in your Sauce-pan, with a
little good Broth, made of a Neck of Beef, put all
the Haricals in but the Liver; when they are enough,
put in a good Deal of Spinage, a little Parfley, and an
Onion, feafon it with Pepper and Salt, and let it ftew on
a flow Fire: You may put in it half a Pound of Prunes,
and thicken it with Crumbs of Bread if you pleafe.

To drefs any Sort of Liver.

CUT the Liver in thin Pieces, and rub it all over
with Eggs; take Crumbs of Bread, fweet Herbs, Onions and Lemon-peel fhred fmall, and ftrew it on it,
feafon it with Pepper and Salt: You may either fry or
broil it, make your Sauce of a little Gravy, thickened
with Butter work'd in Flour, the Juice of a Lemon, a
little Ketchup, and grated Nutmeg.

To roaft a Ham or Gammon of Bacon.

TAKE off the Skin, and lay it to fteep in lukewarm
Water; then lay it in a Pan, pour on it a Mutchkin
of Canary, and let it fteep in it twelve Hours, then
fpit

spit it and paper it over the fat Side; pour the Canary it was foaked in, into the Driping-pan, and bafte it with it all the while it is roafting; when it is roafted enough, pull off the Paper, and drudge it well with Crumbs of Bread, and Parfley fhred fine, brown it well, and fet it to cool. Serve it with green Parfley.

To roaft Pork without the Skin.

TAKE any Joint of Pork not falted, and lay it to the Fire till the Skin may be taken off, then take it up and take off the Skin, then falt it and roaft it, make Sauce for it of Claret, Crumbs of Bread, and a little Water; boil all together, put to it fome Salt, a Piece of Butter, Lemon juice, or Vinegar; when the Pork is roafted flour it, then difh it, and pour the Sauce to it.

To roaft a Breaft of Pork.

TAKE a Fore-quarter of Pork, and cut off the Knuckle, divide the Neck from the Breaft, take out all the Bones, rub it well with Salt, fhread Thyme and Sage fmall; mix with it Nutmeg, Cloves and Mace; ftrew them all over the Meat, then roll it up tight with the Flefh inward; tie it faft together, fpit it long ways and roaft it, put Gravy and Muftard under it.

To broil Pork Steaks.

CUT a Loin or Neck of Pork in thin Steaks, feafon them with Salt and Sage fhred fmall, lay them on the Brander, then feafon the other Side, let the Sauce be beat Butter, Vinegar and Muftard.

To drefs a Pig the French Way.

SPIT your Pig, lay it down to the Fire, and let it roaft till it is thoroughly warm; then take it off the Spit and divide it into twenty Pieces, fet them to ftew in white Wine, and ftrong Broth, feafoned with Nutmeg, Pepper and Salt, two Onions, and two Anchovies cut fmall, and a little Butter and Vinegar; ftew

J them

them all, and when enough difh it in the **Liquor** it was ftewed in, with fliced Orange or Lemon.

A Hog's Head Cheefe Fafhion.

BOIL it till the Bones come out, then feafon it with Pepper, Salt and Cloves, while it is hot put the thin Side of one half, and the thick of the other together; put a Cloth over and under it in a fmall Broth Difh, and lay a Weight on it as broad as the Head is, till it is cold, then take it out of the Cloth; you may fend it whole to the Table, or in Slices. It is to be eaten with Muftard and Vinegar, and Onion, if you pleafe.

Pork Brawn.

. GET a Fore-quarter of the beft and firmeft Pork you can get, cut off the Shank and bone it, falt it with a quarter of an Ounce of Salt-petre, and half an Ounce of Peter falt, two Penny worth of Cochineal; pound them and mix them with a little Salt and brown Sugar, then lay it on a Table with a Weight upon it for four Days, then wipe it dry and roll it up hard, and bind it with broad Tape; put it in boiling Water, and let it boil four Hours, ftill keeping the Pot full of Water, if it is large, it will take five Hours boiling.

In Imitation of Brawn.

BOIL a Set of Nolts Feet very tender, then take a Piece of Pork, boil it near enough; then put the Flefh of the Feet in the Middle of the Pork, let both be boiled with Salt; roll it up tight, and put Tapes about it, boil it till it is tender; when cold put it in Soufe.

A Pig in Jelly.

CUT it in Quarters, and lay it in a Stew pan with two Calves Feet, and the Pig's Feet, put in a Pint of Rhenifh Wine, the Juice of four Lemons, and fome of the Rind, and one *Englifh* Quart of Water; feafon it with Nutmeg, Salt and Mace, ftove it gently for two
Hours,

Hours; let it ſtand till cold, then clear the Jelly; and when it is almoſt cold, put it on the Pig; you may cut the Pig into any Shape you pleaſe, and pour the Jelly over it.

To dreſs a Loin of Pork with Onions.

PUT a Loin of Pork to roaſt, and put twenty ſmall Onions in the Driping-pan under the Pork; let the Fat drop on them, when the Pork is nigh enough put the Onions into the Sauce-pan. Let them ſimmer over the Fire a Quarter of an Hour, ſhaking them well, then pour out all the Fat; ſhake in a little Flour, a Spoonful of Vinegar, and two Tea Spoonfuls of Muſtard, give them a Boil. Lay the Pork in the Diſh, and the Onions in a Sauce Boat.

To roaſt a Quarter of young Pig, Lamb Faſhion.

CUT the Pig in Quarters, and take off the Skin, ſcore it in the Middle with a little Blood, roaſt it a light brown, it will eat like Lamb, with Spearmint, Sugar and Vinegar. The other Part of the Pig you may do in Jelly thus: Bone it, and boil it in a ſmall Quantity of Water, with two Penny-worth of Iſinglaſs, whole Pepper, Cloves, Mace, Lemon-peel and Salt: When it is boil'd as tender that you may thruſt a Straw in it, take it out and cut it in Dice; dry it on a Cloth, put a Gill of white Wine, the Juice of a Lemon, and the Whites of two Eggs beaten in the Liquor the Pig was boil'd in, and run it thro' a Jelly Bag Pleaſe put your Pig that you cut in Dice in a Bowl; and when the Jelly is almoſt cold, pour it over them.

A Pig Rolliand.

BONE it, leaving the Head whole, and rub it over with Eggs; ſeaſon it with Pepper, Salt and Nutmeg, and lay over it ſome Forc'd meat. Then roll it up, and either roaſt, bake, or ſtove it. You may cut it in four Pieces, and ſend the Head in the Middle: Make the

Sauce

Sauce of the Brains, and Gravy, Butter, Vinegar, and chopped Sage if you like it.

To make Bologna Sausages.

TAKE a Pound of Bacon, fat and lean together, a Pound of Beef, a Pound of Veal, a Pound of Pork, and a Pound of Beef Sewet, chop them very fine, sweet Herbs and Sage shred very small, and Pepper; and, to season it pretty high, get a large Gut and fill it, boil the Water, and prick the Gut for fear of bursting. Boil it softly an Hour, then lay it on clean Straw to dry, it will keep good a Year in a dry Place.

To fry Sausages with Apples or Potatoes.

TAKE a Pound of Sausages and six Apples or Potatoes, cut them as thick as a Crown, fry them with Sausages a light brown, dish them up hot, stew'd Cabbage, and fried Sausages, or Pease Pudding and Sausages eat very well.

Oister Sausages.

TAKE a Pound of the Lean of a Leg of Mutton, and two Pound of Beef Sewet, shred very fine, three half Mutchkins of Oisters, shread them likewise, mix these with some of the Oister Liquor, Pepper, Salt, Cloves, Mace, and three raw Eggs, and make them up as you use them, and fry them in Butter.

Oxford Sausages.

CHOP the Lean of a Leg of Veal or Mutton, with four Pound of Beef Sewet, or Butter; season it with Pepper, Salt, Cloves and Mace; pound them well, with five or six Eggs, and as you use them roll them out long-ways with Flour; when you fry them boil the Butter, and then put in the Sausages; fry them a light brown, this will serve for Forc'd-meat Balls.

A

A Soufe for Brawn.

BOIL Wheat Brawn and Salt very well, then ftrain it; and when cold, put in the Brawn: There muft be a good deal of Salt; new boil it every Fortnight.

To make Saufages.

TAKE the tendereft Part of a Leg of Pork, and chop it very fmall; to every Pound of Flefh put a Pound of Hog's Fat, or Beef Sewet; when both is finely chopp'd pound them together in a Mortar; feafon them with Salt, Black and *Jamaica* Pepper; they muft be high feafoned: Let them lye a Day before you put them in the Skins. Let your Skins be very clean, and lye a while in Salt and Water. You may put chopped Sage in them. You may make Mutton the fame Way; but put no Sage in them.

Pig's Petty-toes.

WHEN the Pig is opened, get the Draught and Feet clean, and boil them; then get a little Gravy, and a Bit of Butter and Flour, an Onion, and two or three Leaves of Sage minc'd fmall: Cut the Feet in two, and mince the Draught very fmall, feafon it with Pepper and Salt, boil them together, and ferve it up; it muft be a young Pig's Draught.

To roaft a Pig's Haflet.

CUT it afunder and wafh it well; ftuff the Heart with Crumbs of Bread, fhred Sage, Onion, Parfley and fweet Marjoram, Pepper, Salt and *Jamaica* Pepper; work all this up with a little Butter: Spit them, and ftrew Crumbs of Bread, and fome of the fame Seafoning all over it, but firft rub it with an Egg to make it ftick. Roll the Caul, or a buttered Paper over it, and tye it faft, but when you think it done take off the Paper. It takes two Hours to roaft it. Serve it up with Gravy and Butter, and a little Sage, with a Drop of Vinegar in it.

To make a Ragoo of Tripes.

WHEN boiled, cut them in Bits, put them in a Stew-pan with a very little Water, and feason them with Pepper, Salt and a Blade of Mace, with fhred Parfley and Onions; when tenderly ftewed, put to them a little Cream and Butter work'd in Flour; ferve them up with Sippets under them: You may do Cow Heels the fame Way, but inftead of Cream put Muftard.

To drefs a large Pig's Feet and Ears.

BOIL them tender in Salt and Water, then cut your Ears in thin Slices, and your Feet in Quarters: When boiled, fry them, and for their Sauce, get melted Butter, Onions, Parfley, Vinegar and Muftard; boil your Parfley and Onions in your Butter, chopping them firft.

To make a Ragoo of Mufhrooms.

WASH and dry them, put them in a clofs covered Sauce-pan, with a little Pepper, Salt and a Blade of Mace: Put three Spoonfuls of Water in them, put them on a flow Fire. They take a great while ftewing; when tender, thicken them with a little Butter work'd in Flour; and before you fend them to the Table, put two Spoonfuls of white Wine in them, and half an one of Vinegar or Lemon.

To make a Ragoo of Kidneys.

TAKE them, and cut them in thin Slices, flour them and fry them in Butter: When enough, pour in a little Gravy or Water, feafon them with Pepper, Salt and fhred Onion and Parfley, with a little Vinegar: You may put in a little Ketchup. Give them but three Boils after you feafon them.

To ragoo a Breaft of Veal.

STUFF it with Forc'd-meat between the Flefh and the Bones, and lard it with Bacon if you like it,
then

then half roaft it, and put it in a Stew-pan with Gravy, and ftove it till it is enough, then put in Forc'd meat Balls, Mufhrooms, Truffles, Morels and Oifters; feafon it with Pepper, Salt, Mace and Nutmeg; the Truffles and Morels muft be wafhed and half boiled before you put them in; thicken it with brown'd Butter and Flour, put in a Glafs of white Wine and fome Lemon Juice.

A Ragoo of Lambs Stones and Sweet-breads.

BLANCH them in boiling Water, then wipe them dry, and fry them a light brown; then put them in a Stew-pan with fome good Gravy, Pepper, Salt, and an Onion ftuffed with Cloves, Mufhrooms and Truffles; let them fimmer over a gentle Fire, then put in a Piece of Butter rolled in Flour, a little white Wine and Lemon Juice, and boil them, keeping them ftirring all the Time to mix the Butter. You may cut them in Slices, and parboil them with blanched Cocks Combs, and not fry them, but tofs them with the fame Ingredients as before; or you may dip them in Batter, made of a little Ale, Flour and two Eggs; then fry them, and difh them with nothing but fried Parfley over them, beat Butter, and Juice of Orange in a Cup.

To ragoo a Neck of Veal.

CUT it in Steaks, feafon it with Pepper, Salt, Cloves and Mace; lard them with Bacon, dip them in Eggs, make up a Sheet of Cap Paper fquare, and pin the four Corners an Inch high, butter it, fet it on the Grid-iron on a flow Fire, put in the Meat, let it do leifurely, keeping it turning and bafting; when it is enough, have ready Gravy, Mufhrooms, Pickles, Forc'd-meat Balls, and fried Oifters, feafon it pretty high, lay the Veal in the Difh, and pour the Sauce over it: Put into it white Wine and Lemon Juice.

To ragoo Venison.

LARD a Piece of Venison with Bacon, well season-ed with Pepper and Salt, fry it a light Brown, then stew it two Hours in Broth or boiling Water, and some Claret, season it with Pepper, Salt, Nutmeg and Le-mon-peel, thicken it with Butter work'd in Flour, put a little Lemon Juice and Capers in it.

A Ragoo of Livers.

GET the Livers of Fowls, Turkeys or Geese, take off the Gall, blanch them; then put them in a Stew-pan, with as much Gravy as will cover them, a Bit of Butter rolled in Flour, Pepper, Salt, Oisters and Ketchup: Let them stew twelve Minutes if large, but six if small. You may put in Crumbs of Bread, and an Onion shred small.

To ragoo a green Goose.

CUT the Goose in two, put it in a Stew pan with some Butter, sliced Onions, Lemon, Pepper, Cloves and Salt. You may put in a Bunch of sweet Herbs, put it on a slow Fire, stir and turn it often, then make a Ragoo of green Pease, a little Butter, and some good Gravy, Pepper, Salt and Nutmeg; shake in a little Flour; dish your Goose, and pour the Pease on it.

A Ragoo for a Duck à la Braise.

HALF roast the Duck, and carbonade it, then make a Ragoo of Sweet-breads, fat Fowls Livers, Cocks Combs, Mushrooms if in Season, Asparagus Tops, Ar-tichoke Bottoms and Truffles, all blanched and half boiled; then stew them in Gravy, seasoned with Pepper, Salt, Cloves, and shred Shalots: Put the Duck in the Middle of the Dish, and pour the Ragoo over it.

To ragoo Pigeons.

LARD your Pigeons, cut some of them in two, season them with Salt, Pepper, Cloves and Mace; then
brown

brown some Butter and Flour, and put in your Pigeons, and brown them; then put in as much Gravy as will cover them, with a Faggot of sweet Herbs, and let them stew on a slow Fire; when they are enough stewed, take out the Herbs, and put in Shalots, Anchovies, Oisters and Mushrooms. You may put about them, when they are dished, roasted Larks, or any small Birds.

A Ragoo of a Calf's Head.

BOIL it, and cut it in long small Pieces, an Inch long, and the Breadth of your Finger; put them in a Stew-pan with a little Gravy, Truffles, Morels, Oisters, Artichoke Bottoms in Slices, Juice of Lemon, Pepper, Salt and Mace; thicken it with Butter and Flour, boil it, and put white Wine in it.

To make a Ragoo of Onions.

GIVE them a Scald, then drain them, and put Gravy, Pepper, and Salt to them: Let them simmer on a slow Fire a good while, then put to them a Piece of Butter rolled in Flour. They may be eaten with any roasted or boiled Meat.

A Ragoo of stuffed Cucumbers.

TAKE as many Cucumbers as will fill your Dish, pare them, and scoop out the Seeds, blanch them with boiling Water, then put them in cold Water, stuff them with Veal, Beef, and Sewet shred very small; season it with Pepper, Salt, Onions, Lemon-peel and Spice. Thicken it with Butter and Flour.

To fry Tripe Ragoo.

CUT them into small Pieces, dip them in the Yolks of Eggs, and strew on them Crumbs of Bread; fry them of a brown Colour, drain them from the Fat, and send them up hot with Butter and Mustard in a Sauce Boat.

K

To

To roaſt Tripe.

CUT them in ſquare Pieces, make a Ragoo of Forc'd meat, Crumbs of Bread, Butter, Pepper, Salt and Nutmeg, and the Yolks of two Eggs; ſpread it on the Tripe, roll them up tight, and tye your Rolls on the Spit, flour and baſte it. Serve them with melted Butter and ſliced Orange.

Tripes the Poliſh Way.

CUT the Tripes in Pieces, and ſtrew them with Crumbs, Parſley, green Onions, Pepper and Salt; then put into the Stew-pan a Lump of Butter, and when it is brown, put in the Tripes. Let them ſtew till they are of a good Colour; the Sauce is Butter and Lemon.

To boil Tripes.

CUT them in Pieces, and boil them in Salt and Water till they are tender. You may either ſend them in their own Broth, with Onions and Pepper in it, or boil Onions and chop them; then put them in beat Butter, and ſend it in a Boat; ſome Leeks, Parſley and Onions with them.

To make a Ragoo of Palates and Eyes.

WHEN they are cut out of the Ox or Cow's Head, take the Black out of the Eyes, then blanch them in ſcalding Water, and blanch and ſkin the Palates, boil them in Salt and Water, when boiled cut your Palates in thin Slices, and your Eyes in round ones, but let them both be very thin, put them both in your Stew-pan with ſome good Gravy, an Onion ſtuffed with Cloves, a Bunch of ſweet Herbs, Pepper, and Salt; ſtew them well, then take out your Herbs and put in a little Ketchup, brown ſome Butter and Flour, then pour all in, keeping it ſtirring all the Time; put a little Lemon Juice or Vinegar in it before you ſerve it up, and Forc'd-meat Balls, Oiſters, and white Wine.

To make a Ragoo of Sheeps Tongues and Sweet-breads or Kernels.

BOIL your Tongues and blanch them; cut them in very thin Slices, and your Kernels in Dice; stew them in Gravy with boiled Artichoke Bottoms cut in Quarters; then season them with Salt, Pepper, Cloves and Anchovies; brown your Butter and Flour, put them in it, keeping them stirring all the Time; put Lemon Juice, or a very little Vinegar in it: You may put Truffles and Morels in it, if you please.

To make a Ragoo of Truffles and Morels.

BOIL them in Water, when boiled strain the Water they are boiled in, and pick and clean them; put them and their own Liquor in a Stew-pan, with Butter, and Flour, Pepper, Salt, Cloves, Anchovies, a whole Onion, and a little Gravy, when they are stewed well, put a little white Wine and the Juice of a Lemon in it: Serve them up garnished with Forc'd-meat Balls and sliced Lemon.

To make Brain Cakes.

BOIL and blanch the Calf's Brains, chop some of them, and mix them with Crumbs of Bread, Spice, Salt, the Grate of a Lemon, sweet Herbs shred small, and an Egg; then cut in Pieces what you leave, and rub them with an Egg; strew Flour on them, fry them all in a Pan of boiling Liquor; put in the chopped Brains in Spoonfuls, the other in Lumps; garnish your Heads with these.

To make Veal Cutlets.

CUT a Neck of Veal in single Bones, and rub them over with Eggs; strew on them grated Bread, Salt, Pepper, Nutmeg, shred Parsley, Shalots, and Lemon-peel; mix them with the Crumbs of Bread; brander them on buttered Papers, or you may do them in the Oven on Tin Plates: For your Sauce, get a little Gra-

vy,

vy, a Bit of Butter work'd in Flour, a little white Wine, feafon it with Nutmeg and Salt; put in it a chopped Anchovy, and fome Mufhrooms, if you have them; garnifh your Difh with Pickles and fliced Lemon; put a little Lemon Juice in your Sauce. You may do Mutton or Lamb the fame Way.

To mince Fowl, Veal or Lamb.

WHEN your Fowl or Flefh is half roafted, mince it fmall; put it in your Stew-pan with a little white Gravy, a Piece of Butter worked in Flour, a Blade of Mace, a little Pepper and Salt, a whole Onion, the Rind of a Lemon, and a little of the Juice, a minced Anchovy, fome Mufhrooms likeways. Give it but one or two Boils, for Fear of making the Meat hard; garnifh it with fliced Lemon: Take out the Onion and Lemon-peel, before you fend it to the Table.

To fry Veal Sweet-breads.

HAVING larded them with Bacon, run a Skewer through them, or a Spit, and roaft them till they are brown; then lay them in a Difh, and put Gravy under them.

To farce Veal Sweet-breads.

SCALD the Sweet-breads, and lard them with Bacon, make a Hole in them, and ftuff it with good Forc'd-meat, don't make the Hole quite through, then bake them in a Pan; make a Ragoo of Mufhrooms, Truffles, Artichoke Bottoms and Cocks-combs, and Forc'd-meat Balls, and a little good Gravy thicken'd with the Yolks of Eggs: Difh the Sweet-breads, and put a little Juice of Orange, Salt, Mace and Nutmeg, in the Ragoo, then pour it about them: You may at another Time blanch fome Sweet-breads, and cut them in Slices; flour them and fry them, and put beat Butter, with Gravy, Nutmeg and Orange about them.

Rolled

Rolled Fricandoes of Veal.

CUT Slices of a Leg of Veal, beat them, lard them, lay them on the Table, the larded Side downwards: Cover them the Thickness of a Crown, with Forc'd-meat made of Veal, Beef Sewet or Marrow; season it with Pepper, Salt, Nutmeg and Lemon-peel, and a chopped Anchovy: Put Eggs to bind them, roll them up, and you may do them in the Oven, or fry them in a Pan of boiling Fat. You may either put a Ragoo of Sweet breads and Palates under them, or Gravy, and the Juice of a Lemon. Be sure to drain the Fat well from them.

To roast a Calf's Liver.

LARD your Liver with Bacon fastened on the Spit, roast it at a gentle Fire; baste it well, and serve it up with beat Butter, Gravy, and a little Vinegar. A Calf's Liver brander'd gets the same Sauce.

To broil any Sort of Midriffs.

TAKE the largest and freshest you can get, clean and scald them well, stuff them with Forc'd-meat, or with Onion, Sage, Pepper and Salt; then sew them up, and lay them to broil on a moderate Fire, serve them up with Gravy, with or without Claret.

CHAP. IV.

To make Pyes and Pasties, &c.

To make a Venison Pasty.

BONE and season your Venison, and let it lye all Night in Seasoning, boil the Bones that come out of it into good Gravy, put it into the Pasty-pan, with good Puff Paste about it; it takes a great while to bake it.

When

When it comes out of the Oven shake it; and if there is not Gravy enough in it, put in more; if it is to be eaten hot, not elfe, Pepper and Salt is the Seasoning.

To make a Mutton Pasty as good as Venison.

BONE your Fore quarter of Mutton, and put it in Steep in Claret and its own Blood, a Mutchkin of each, let it lye all Night, season it with Pepper and Salt; put it in your Dish with all that is steep'd in about it: Cover it with Puff Paste, bake it two Hours in a hot Oven. When it comes out of the Oven, shake the Dish; and if it wants Gravy put it in. You may put Blood and Claret in a Venison Pasty, if you please.

To make a Pigeon Pye.

CUT off the Pinions and Feet, draw them, and chop the Liver and Giffart, mix it with Crumbs of Bread, chopped Parsley, Lemon-peel and Onion work'd up with a Piece of Butter, Pepper and Salt; season your Pye with Pepper and Salt; put the Stuffing in their Bellies, lay them in the Dish on their Breasts, and put a little Butter on them; put the Pinions in the Dish with them. Cover the Pye with Puff Paste, so bake it in a quick Oven. You may eat it either hot or cold; you may make it without Stuffing if you please.

To make a Lamb Pye.

CUT your Lamb in middling Pieces, season it with Pepper, Salt and Cloves: Put it in your Dish with hard Yolks of Eggs and Artichoke Bottoms, and a little Gravy or Water. Cover it with Puff Paste: You may put in Raisins and Prunes if you please.

To make a Veal Florentine.

CUT your Veal in small Pieces, season it with Pepper, Salt, Cloves and Mace: Put them in your Dish with Currants and Raisins, a little Bit of Butter, and the Squeeze of a Lemon, and a Gill of Water. Cover
your

your Dish with Puff Paste; and when it comes out of the Oven, have a Caudle of a Gill of Gravy, a Gill of white Wine, a little Nutmeg, thickened with the Yolks of two Eggs, put a little Sugar in it, and pour it in your Pye. This Caudle will serve for any sweet Pye. Shake the Dish after it is in it.

To make a Chicken Pye.

SCALD your Chickens, and cut them in Quarters, wash them very clean; season them with Pepper, Salt, Cloves and Mace; put them in your Dish with Forc'd-meat Balls, Yolks of hard Eggs, and Artichoke Bottoms. You may make it without this if you please; put a little Butter and Gravy You may put Fruit in it, if you like it sweet, and make a Caudle for it as above. You may leave the Chickens whole if you please.

To make a Calf's Foot Pye.

BOIL your Feet and mince them with a little Beef or Mutton Sewet, and some Apples shred small, a little Cinnamon and Mace pounded, some Currants well washed and picked; put them all in a Dish with Puff Paste over them, three Quarters of an Hour bakes them: Then have a Caudle of Cherry, Nutmeg and Sugar thickened with Eggs; the Oven must be no hotter than will bake the Paste. You may make a Chadren Pye the same Way. Put a Gill of Brandy in it.

To make an Eel Pye.

CUT off the Head and Fins, and cut them two Inches long; season them with black and *Jamaica* Pepper, Cloves and Salt. Put them in your Dish, with some Butter and Crumbs of Bread, a little white Wine and Lemon Juice, and Gravy or Water, half a Mutchkin of either. Cover it with Puff Paste.

To make a Goose Pye.

BONE and season it with Pepper and Salt: If your Goose be very fat, bone a Turkey or a Pair of Fowls, and put in with it. You may either raise it or put it in a Dish: It is to be eat cold. It takes a great while to bake it.

To make a Trout Pye.

CUT off the Fins and Heads, season them with black and *Jamaica* Pepper, Mace and Salt, put some Butter in the Bottom of your Dish, then your Trouts; put Gravy and a little Claret in it : Cover it with Puff Paste. When the Paste is baked, they are enough. They are good hot or cold. You may bake Carp or Pike the same Way.

To make a Mutton Steak Pye.

CUT a Neck of Mutton in single Bones, season it with black and *Jamaica* Pepper and Salt, lay them in your Dish with Artichoke Bottoms if you have them, put Gravy or Water in the Dish, and a little chopped Shalot. You may make a Beef Steak Pye the same Way. Put some Oisters in it if you please, and hard Yolks of Eggs.

To make a Lobster or Shrimp Pye.

BOIL your Lobsters and Shrimps, take off the Shells, cut the Lobsters in large Pieces, the Shrimps whole. Put Butter in the Bottom of your Dish; season them with Pepper, Mace, Salt and Nutmeg. Put a little Gravy, Oister Liquor, white Wine, and the Juice of a Lemon in it. You may put both in the Pye if you please. Put Puff Paste on it. A very little bakes it.

To make an Oister Pye.

GET the largest Oisters you can, wash them clean in their own Liquor, and give them a Blanch;

get

get alſo half a Dozen Sweet-breads, and cut them in Pieces, put Gravy and Butter in the Diſh, then lay a Lair of each, till your Pye is full, and a Lair of Forc'd meat Balls; ſeaſon it with Pepper, Salt and Cloves; put a little Oiſter Liquor in it, and ſome Lemon Juice. When baked, put in a Caudle of Cherry, the Grate of a Nutmeg, thickened with the Yolks of two Eggs. You may put the Yolks of hard Eggs in it if you like them, and Artichoke Bottoms, or Truffles and Morels.

To make a Skirret Pye.

BOIL and peel your Skirrets, put them in the Diſh, with Butter on the Bottom of it, and a few Crumbs of Bread; cover them almoſt with Cream, Nutmeg and Mace pounded, ſweeten it with Sugar, cover it with Puff Paſte: When it comes out of the Oven, pour in a Caudle made of white Wine, Sugar, and the Grate of a Nutmeg, thickened with the Yolks of two Eggs.

To make minc'd Pyes.

BOIL a large Ox Tongue, blanch it, and chop it ſmall, put double the Quantity of Beef Sewet, as you have of Tongue, and the double of Fruit, Currants waſhed and picked clean, the Raiſins ſton'd and minc'd, your Sewet minc'd very fine, and half a Dozen Apples minc'd; ſeaſon it with Cloves, Mace, Nutmeg, Lemon-peel, Cinnamon, and a little Sugar and Salt: Put half a Mutchkin of Brandy in it: When you put it in your Pan, put Puff Paſte over and under it: You may put candyed Citron, Lemon and Orange-peel, if you pleaſe.

To make an Apple Pye.

PARE and quarter your Apples, take out the Cores, put Sugar, beat Cinnamon, and the Grate of a Lemon in it, and the Bigneſs of an Egg of Butter: If you pleaſe you may put Marmelade of Orange or Quince in it: Cover it with Puff Paſte. A Pear Pye

L

is made the fame Way, but put the Juice of a Lemon in it : and if your Apples are dry, put Lemon Juice in it: When either is cold, you may pour Cream over them, if you pleafe.

To make a Beef Steak Pye.

CUT a very tender fat Piece of Beef in thin Slices, beat it with the Rolling-pin, feafon it with Pepper, Salt, and Cloves, ftrew it with a little chopped Shalot, fill your Difh, and cover it with Puff Pafte. When it is baked, put in a little Gravy: You may put Oifters in the Pye if you pleafe, and if you do, put in with your Gravy a Glafs of white Wine. Make a Mutton chopp'd Pye the fame Way: You may put in it Forc'd-meat, Truffles, Morels, and Artichoke Bottoms, but put them between the Lairs of the Steaks.

To make a Goofe-berry Pye.

IF your Goofe-berries are very young, put them in a Stew-pan, and ftove them with Sugar, when cold, put them in your Difh, and nick the Pafte that covers them. When the Pafte is baked, they are enough: You may fend them to the Table as they are, or cream them. If you cream them, cut off the Lid, and pour it on them: If it is thin, boil it, and thicken it with the Yolks of two Eggs, and fweeten it to your Tafte, but take Care it is not curdled: When it is cold pour it on, cut the Lid in Pieces, and ftick it round the Pye.

To make a Hare Pye.

CUT your Hare in Pieces, break the Bones, and feafon it to your Tafte, with Pepper, Salt, Cloves and Mace; lay it in your Difh with Slices of Butter and Lemon Juice : Cover it with Puff Pafte.

To make a Gibblet Pye.

WHEN your Gibblets are well fcalded and blanch-ed, break the Bones, and feafon them with Pepper, Salt,

Cloves,

Cloves and Mace; put them to ſtew in as much Water as will cover them; ſet them on a ſlow Fire, and
when they are tender ſet them to cool: If you can
get the Blood, make a Pudding in the Skin of the Neck
thus: Strain the Blood, and put in it a little Sewet,
ſhred ſmall, ſome Crumbs of Bread, a Gill of Cream,
Pepper, Salt, Nutmeg, a little ſweet Herbs ſhred ſmall,
and an Onion; lay the Pudding in the Middle of the
Diſh, and the Gibblets round it; pour the Broth they
were boiled in over them; let them be well ſeaſoned:
Cover the Diſh with Puff Paſte.

To make a Lark Pye, or any ſmall Birds.

TAKE the Larks and ſeaſon them with Pepper,
Salt and Mace; ſtuff them with Forc'd–meat, and lay
them in the Diſh with Puff Paſte about the Diſh, the
Yolks of hard Eggs, Artichoke Bottoms, and a Lair of
Forc'd meat; put ſome Butter over them, and cover
it with Puff Paſte: When baked make a Caudle of Gravy, a Glaſs of white Wine, a little Bit of Butter worked in Flour, and the Grate of a Nutmeg, boil it and
keep it ſtirring, till the Rawneſs is off the Flour; then
pour it in the Pye, then ſhake the Pye, and ſend it up
hot: You may make it without Forc'd-meat or Artichoke Bottoms, the ſame Way.

To make a Muir-fowl or Partridge Pye.

SEASON them with Pepper, Salt, Cloves and
Mace, very well, take Cabbage Lettice that is whole,
and blanch them; lay one between every Fowl, chop
a little Sholot, and ſtrew it on the Lettice, with a little
of the Seaſoning as before: Cover the Diſh with Puff
Paſte, cut it in the prettieſt Faſhion you can: When
it is baked make a Sauce of two Gills of Claret, a little
Gravy, an Anchovy and a little Nutmeg; pour it in
the Pye and ſhake it, ſo ſend it up hot.

A

A Partridge Pye.

TAKE your Patridges and feafon them with Pepper, Salt, Cloves and Mace; then take fix Cabbage Lettice, boil them four Minutes, fqueeze the Water well from them, put Puff Pafte in the Difh, and lay in the Partridges, with a Lettice between every one, and Saufages: Firft fry them a little, and put in a Glafs of white Wine, and a Piece of Butter; cover it with a thick Pafte; bake it two Hours. For the Sauce have Gravy well feafoned, put it in the Top of the Pye, with a Funnel, and fhake the Pye. You may put in Claret inftead of white Wine, if you pleafe.

To make a Pye of Mutton and Potatoes.

TAKE a Breaft of Mutton, and cut it in Steaks, feafon it with Pepper and Salt, lay a Lair of Mutton and a Lair of Potatoes, fcraped and fliced, then a Lair of fliced Onions, fo go on till you fill the Difh, feafon them between every Lair; cover it with Puff Pafte two Hours; bake it, put a Piece of fweet Butter in it and Gravy, when it comes out of the Oven.

To make a Pye of Kernels and Artichokes.

BLANCH the Kernels, and boil the Artichoke Bottoms; boil Eggs hard, take out the Yolks, put Butter in the Bottom of the Difh, then the Kernels, then a Lair of Artichoke Bottoms, and a Lair of the Yolks of Eggs: So fill the Difh in Lairs, feafon them with Pepper, Salt, Cloves, Mace and Lemon peel; put Butter over them; then cover it with Puff Pafte, have ready a Ragoo of Truffles, Morels, Gravy, with a little brown'd Butter and Flour, a Glafs of white Wine, an Onion ftuffed with Cloves, and the Rind of a Lemon; boil them, then cut off the Top of the Pye, and pour your Ragoo on it, put on the Top again, and fend it up hot.

T

To make an Apple Pye with Potatoes.

PEEL and slice the Apples, half boil the Potatoes, pare and slice them in Lairs in the Dish with Sugar, Cinnamon, grated Lemon-peel, and a Piece of Butter. You may put Currants, Raisins, and candyed Orange : cover the Pye and bake it. Send it up hot.

To make an Apple Pye with Chesnuts and Almonds.

PARE and quarter the Apples, scald the Chesnuts, and take off the Skin, blanch the Almonds; lay them in Lairs in the Dish : Put in candyed Orange and Lemon peel, and fine Sugar ; put in a Bit of Butter : When the Apples are full ripe, put in the Juice of a Lemon. Cover it with Puff Paste : It is to be eaten either hot or cold. If cold, cream it.

To make a white Fricasey of Lamb.

CUT a Neck and Breast of Lamb in middling small Pieces, put them in hot Water to blanch, then put them in cold Water; when they are blanch'd put them in a closs cover'd Stew-pan, with a Mutchkin of Water, a Bunch of sweet Herbs, a whole Onion stuffed with Cloves, the Rind of a Lemon, and a Blade of Mace : Let them stew on a gentle Fire till the Meat is enough ; then put in a good Piece of Butter work'd in Flour, and a Gill of thick Cream, keep it stirring all the while it is on the Fire. After you put in the Butter, when the Rawness is off the Flour, put in a Glass of Sherry, and the Squeeze of a Lemon. Don't make it too sour, or put it on the Fire after ; salt it to your Taste : Take out the Onion and Herbs, so serve it up. Garnish it with Lemons and Mushrooms.

To make a white Fricasey of Mushrooms.

WASH the little white Mushrooms in Milk and Water, put them down to boil in a little Water and a Blade of Mace, a little white Pepper, with a whole Shalot. When they are tender, put to them a little

Cream,

Cream, and a Bit of Butter worked in Flour. When you put them down to boil, put but a very little Watter in it, and let them be very clofs covered: Juft as you are fending them up, put a little white Wine and a very little Lemon Juice, keeping it ftirring all the Time.

To fricafey Tripes or Cow-heels.

LET them lye in Soufe till they are a little four, then take them out and dry them with a Cloth; make a Batter of Eggs and Flour, and dip them in it, put them in your Pan to fry when the Liquor is boiling hot. The Sauce for them is Butter and Muftard.

To make a white Fricafey of Chickens.

CUT your Chickens in Quarters, then cut every Quarter in two, put them in a Pan with Water to co ver them, and give them a Boil or two; then put them in cold Water, take off the Skin and blanch them; put them in a clofs covered Pan with Muh-rooms, and Truffles with them, a Piece of Butter, a little Flour, a little Salt, a Blade of Mace, a whole O-nion ftuffed with Cloves, a whole Anchovy, and the Rind of a Lemon; fhake the Pan till the Flour mixes, put them on a flow Fire. When they are boil'd enough put in a Gill of thick fweet Cream, and juft as you are going to fend it up put in a little white Wine, and a very little Juice of Lemons. You may beat the Yolks of two Eggs, and mix them with the Sauce to thicken it, but take great Care not to curdle them. You may make it without Muhrooms, or Truffles, if you pleafe.

To make a Fricafey of Rabbits.

CUT them in Quarters and blanch them as above, then boil them; when they are enough throw off the Water, and put to them fome white Gravy, Anchovy, an Onion ftuffed with Cloves, Pepper, Salt, Mace, and the Rind of a Lemon, a good Piece of Butter work'd in Flour, and a Bunch of fweet Herbs. Let them boil

a

a good while, then put in a little good Cream, and juſt as you are going to diſh it, put in a little Sherry, and a very little Lemon Juice.

To make a brown *Fricaſey* of *Chickens* or *Rabbits.*

BROWN your Butter and Flour, then put in Gravy, ſhake it that it does not go to Lumps; put in your Meat with Pepper, Cloves, and *Jamaica* Pepper, an Onion and Lemon peel, put a little Ketchup and the Juice of a Lemon; ſalt it to your Taſte. Garniſh them with Lemon.

To fricaſey *Kernels* and *Oiſters.*

BLANCH the Kernels, cut them in Dice, and ſcald the Oiſters, pick and waſh them clean in their own Liquor, then put them both in a Stew-pan, with a little white Gravy, and ſome of the Oiſter Liquor, ſtrained very clear, an Onion ſtuffed with Cloves, Mace and Lemon-peel, with a Piece of Butter rolled in Flour, and a Gill of Cream: Give them eight or ten Boils, then ſhake in a little white Wine and Lemon Juice, but don't put it on the Fire. After the Wine and Juice goes in, take out the Lemon-peel and Onion, then ſerve it up.

A white *Fricaſey* of *Cows Palates.*

BOIL, blanch and ſkin them, then cut them in Shaves the croſs Way, as broad as your Finger; put them in a Stew pan with Muſhrooms, Truffles, white Gravy, three whole Shalots, white Pepper, two Anchovies, Salt and Mace, a Piece of Butter, a little Flour, and a Gill of Cream; put them on a flow Fire, and when they are very tender, take them off, and put in a Glaſs of white Wine, and Lemon Juice. Don't put them on the Fire after. Put Sippets in the Diſh under them.

A

A white Fricasey of Lambs Stones, Kernels, and Cocks Combs.

BLANCH and boil the Cocks Combs till they are tender, blanch the Kernels, nick the Skin of the Lambs Stones, and turn them out of the Skins; then blanch them, and put them all in a Pan with Veal Gravy, whole white Pepper, Mace, Salt, and a whole Onion; stew them on a slow Fire, then put in a little thick Cream, the Grate of a Lemon, and a Bit of sweet Butter; take it up, and mix it with the Yolks of two Eggs well beaten; then put it on the Fire till it is scalding hot, then put in a little white Wine, and send it away.

A white Fricasey of Oisters.

SCALD them, and wash them in their own Liquor, then put them in a Pan with some white Gravy, and some of their own Liquor, Cream, white Pepper, Mace and Salt, a good Piece of Butter rolled in Flour, a whole Onion, and the Rind of a Lemon: Give them a boil or two, then dish them on Sippets. You may make a white Fricasey of Cockles or Scollops the same Way.

To fry Chickens, Lamb or Veal.

CUT the Chickens in Quarters, and your Lamb or Veal in small Joints, put them to stew in as much Water as will cover them; set them on a slow Fire, in a closs covered Pan. When they are almost enough, put in a good Handful of Parsley, and a few green Onions, then a little before you take them up, put in four or five Eggs, with pounded Pepper, Salt and Mace, then dish them up.

A white Fricasey of Skirrets or Parsnips.

BOIL, blanch and skin them, then put them in a Pan, with as much Milk as will cover them, with a good Piece of Butter, white Pepper, Mace pounded, and two whole Onions: Boil them on a slow Fire,
then

then thicken them with the Yolks of two or three Eggs. The Parſnips and Skirrets muſt be cut an Inch long. Don't let them boil after you put in the Eggs: You may do Potatoes the ſame Way: Take out the Onions, and ſerve them up.

To ſtew Chickens with Peaſe and Lettices.

TAKE two Chopins of young Peaſe, and three Cabbage Lettices; ſlice the Lettice, and put the Peaſe in a Sauce-pan, with a Mutchkin of good white Gravy, two Chickens truſſed for boiling; rub the Chickens with a Bit of Butter, and put a Piece of Butter in with the Peaſe; put in a Faggot of ſweet Herbs, if you like it, ſeaſon it with Pepper and Salt; put your Chickens in the Middle of your Diſh, and pour the Peaſe over them: You may ſtove Lamb or Ducks the ſame Way.

Boiled Ducks and Onions.

BOIL your Ducks very white, then boil twelve Onions very tender, ſhifting the Water to take off the Taſte; chop them, and draw eight Ounces of Butter, with two Gills of Cream, when it boils, ſtir in the Onions, and a little Salt, lay your Ducks in the Diſh, and pour your Onions over them. Rabbets are done the ſame Way.

To boil a Turkey or Fowls with Sellery.

BOIL your Turkey or Fowls in a Pot of boiling Water, rub Butter and Flour on the Breaſts, and tye them up in a Cloth: You may ſtuff where their Crops were thus: Two Handfuls of Crumbs of Bread, one of Sewet ſhred ſmall, Lemon-peel, Parſley Thyme, ſweet Marjoram, and a little Onion, all ſhred ſmall, ſeaſon it with Pepper, Salt and Nutmeg, wet it with an Egg, and work it together, ſo ſtuff them full: Cut the Sellery about half an Inch long, waſh it clean, and boil it tender, ſtrain it, and put it in as much white Gravy as you want Sauce, with a

M

good

good Piece of Butter work'd in Flour; feafon it with an Onion, ftuffed with Cloves, Pepper, Salt, Mace, Lemon-peel and Nutmeg, boil it well, then take out the Onion and Lemon-peel, and put in a little white Wine and the Juice of half a Lemon. Don't make it too four, you may boil Fowls or Turkeys, with Oifter Sauce to the Meat.

Or this Sauce for Hens or Chickens.

BOIL the Liver and two Eggs hard, chop them fmall, mince Parfley and Lemon-peel; then put them all into beat Butter, with Gravy in it, and a little Lemon Juice.

To roaft a Pig.

WIPE it very dry, and put in the Belly a Cruft of Bread, few it up and fpit it, dredge it very well with Flour, let it have a very good quick Fire, and let it be very faft turned: When you think it is done, wipe off the Flour, and rub it with a Bit of Butter; it will take an Hour and a Quarter to roaft: If large, cut off the Head, and put the Jaws and Ears round the Difh, take out the Brains, and chop them fmall, put them in a little melted Butter and Gravy, Pepper, Salt, a little Sage chopped very fmall, and an Egg boiled and chopped fmall, pour it about the Pig, you may cut it down the Back, or fend it whole, but take out the Bread before you fend it to Table.

To make a white Fricafey Sauce for boiled Fowls, Chickens or Turkeys.

GET white Broth, boil in it the Rind of a Lemon, an Onion ftuffed with Cloves, Mace, whole Pepper and Salt. When it is boiled a while, put in a Gill of Cream and the Yolks of two Eggs beat well together: Keep it ftirring one Way on the Fire: Put a Piece of Butter in it. and juft as it is going to Table, put the Juice of a Lemon and a little white Wine in

it ;

it· Don't make it four : Take out the Onion and Lemon-peel.

To make a Mutton Haricot.

TAKE a Neck or Loin of Mutton, cut them in Steaks, fry them a light brown, but not too much : Put to them some good Broth, a Faggot of sweet Herbs, some diced Carots and Turnips fried, and three small Cabbage Lettices ; stew all well together, with six small Onions, if you like them, season it with Pepper, Salt and Cloves, skim off all the Fat, and dish it up ; there is not to be too much Broth in the Dish.

To roast Chickens in Paste.

TRUSS them as for boiling, stuff them with Forc'd-meat, and make as much Puff Paste as will cover them, then wrap it about the Chickens, with buttered Papers over it, tied at each End : It will take an Hour to roast them : You may put a Ragoo of Truffles and Morels, or Gravy and Mushrooms under them, but take off the Papers. You may do Ducks the same Way.

Chickens and Sellery.

BOIL them white, and make the Sauce thus : Boil the white Ends of Sellery, cut it in Pieces an Inch long, strain it, and put it into beat Butter, with Mushroom and Oister Liquor : Then pour it boiling hot over your Chickens.

Chickens forced with Oisters.

LARD them, then mince Parsley, Truffles, Onions, Mushrooms and Oisters, season it with Pepper, Salt and Mace, put to it the Yolk of an Egg, and a Piece of Butter ; put all this in the Chickens Bellies, then tye both Ends of them, and roast them, put a Ragoo of Oisters about them. You may do Howtoudies, or any white Fowl, the same Way.

Chickens

Chickens with Gravy forc'd.

TAKE Sweet-breads, Mushrooms, Anchovies, Marrow or Butter, Lemon-peel and Chives, all cut small; mix them with Crumbs of Bread, Pepper, Salt and Nutmeg; wet them with an Egg, then raise up the Skin of the Breasts of your Fowls, stuff it and stitch it up again, and lard them: You may fill their Bellies with Oisters, and roast them: Put Gravy under them in the Dish: You may do Pheasants, Turkeys, or what Fowl you please, the same Way.

Chickens Royal.

LARD them, and put good Forc'd-meat in their Bellies, and half roast them; then stove them in good Gravy; make a Ragoo of Mushrooms, Morels, Truffles and Cocks Combs; lay the Chickens in the Dish, and pour the Ragoo over them. You may do Pigeons the same Way.

Chickens with Tongues, Colliflowers and Greens.

BOIL your Chickens in Water and Salt, and your Sheep or Hogs Tongues in another Pot: Skim them, then put the Colliflowers in the Middle, and a Tongue between every Chicken, and the Greens round them, put melted Butter over them.

To boil Chickens and Asparagus.

BOIL the Chickens white with Forc'd meat in their Bellies, cut the Asparagus an Inch long, boil them in Water, then dissolve a little Butter and Salt in Water, with minc'd Parsley, then put in the Asparagus, and boil it better; thicken the Sauce with more Butter, Cream, and a little Flour; season it with white Wine, Nutmeg and Lemon Juice. You may do Sauce for a Fowl the same Way.

To roast young Turkies.

PUT in their Bellies Forc'd-meat, made of their Livers, scalded Oisters, green Onions, Parsley, mince them all, Crumbs of Bread, Salt, Nutmeg, and grated Lemon-peel, mix them all with a Piece of Butter, and a raw Egg: You may either lard them, or roll them in Shaves of Bacon, then paper and roast them; put Gravy in the Dish with them, and Bread-sauce in a Sauce-boat, made thus: Boil some Bread and Water, with a little white Gravy, an Onion stuffed with Cloves, a Blade of Mace, and a little Salt; boil it smooth; put in it a good Lump of Butter, then give it a Boil, take out the Onions before you send it to Table. You may roast Chickens the same Way.

Ducklings à la Mode.

CUT them in Quarters; you may lard the Legs, and brown them off, then stove them in half a Mutchkin of Claret, the same of Gravy, two Shalots, one Anchovy, Pepper and Salt, stove them tender, skim off the Fat, squeeze in a Lemon, so serve it up hot.

Stov'd Ducks the Dutch Way.

TRUSS two Ducks, and lard one, season with Pepper and Salt, and fill the Bellies with small Onions; lay in the Bottom of the Stew-pan half a Pound of Butter; then put in the Ducks, and cover them with sliced Onions: Stove this two Hours gently, keeping it covered all the while; when the Ducks are tender, dish them, shaking a little Vinegar in them.

To dress a Wild-duck with Lemon Juice.

HALF roast the Duck, and carve it; on the Breast put Salt, Pepper, and the Juice of a Lemon in every Incision; lay it on the Breast in a Stew-pan, with a very little Gravy; then turn it and dish it hot in its own Gravy, a Glass of Claret, and two Shalots shred small.

To

To stew Ducks wild or tame.

HALF roast them, then put them in a Stew-pan with two Gills of Claret, and four of Gravy, Pepper, Salt, Shalots or Rockambole; cover them close: You may stuff the Ducks with Forc'd-meat, and make a Ragoo of Sheeps Tongues, Truffles and Morels. Serve them up hot with the Breast up, and the Sauce that they were stewed in about them, with all the Ingredients.

To dress Ducks with Oisters.

TAKE Ducks wild or tame, truss them; make a Ragoo of Sweet-breads, Oisters, Mushrooms, Truffles, Chives, Parsley, Crumbs of Bread, Lemon peel, Pepper, Salt and Eggs; stuff the Ducks with it, and stew them in a close covered Pan, with Gravy, Claret, browned Butter and Flour, Pepper, Salt, Shalot or Onions, put Oisters fried in Butter about them in the Dish, with the Liquor they are stewed in. You do Teal or Widgeon the same Way.

To roast a green Goose.

STUFF it with Bread Forc'd meat; roast it crisp, and let the Sauce be a little Spinage Juice, scalded Goose-berries, a Bit of Butter, Flour, Sugar or Gravy, and green Onions shred small. You may give young Ducks the same Sauce.

To dress a Goose with Onions or Cabbage.

SALT it for a Week, then boil it an Hour, make the Sauce of boiled Onions, chopped small, mixed with melted Butter; or you may boil Cabbage, and chop and stew them in Butter, Pepper and Salt; dish the Goose, and put the Onions or Cabbage about it, with fried Sausages.

To souse a Goose.

BONE your Goose, cut the Flesh square, lay it a steeping in white Wine, Salt, Pepper, Cloves and
Mace,

Mace, for twelve Hours; then take it out, and lay Pieces of Anchovies over it, and Ham minced small; then roll it up hard, and boil it in boiling Water, and the Wine it was steeped in, with Salt, Pepper, and Mace; boil it pretty well, then put it in a Can, and when you are going to serve it up, cut it in two, and lay over it green Parsley.

To dry a Goose.

GET a fat Goose, and salt it well with a Handful of common Salt, a quarter of an Ounce of Salt-petre, a quarter of a Pound of coarse Sugar, mix all together, and rub the Goose very well, let it lye in this Pickle a Fortnight, turning and rubbing it every Day; then roll it in Brawn, then hang it to dry for a Week; it will keep three Months in a dry Place: It eats well cold, or hot, but boil it well in a large Pot full of Water: If eaten hot, send Cabbage, or Greens about it.

To boil a Goose.

PUT it in a Pot with Water, or Broth; let it boil, and skim it clean, put in a little Salt, three sliced Onions, a few Cloves, Mace, Raisins, Currants, and Crumbs of Bread; stew it on a slow Fire, dish it on Sippets, put a little white Wine in it, and put Slices of Lemon, and Barberries over it.

To boil the Gibblets.

BLANCH them, then boil them in Water, Salt, and Mace; serve them up on Sippets, with melted Butter, and scalded Grapes.

To roast a Goose.

STUFF it with boiled Potatoes, and Onions, chopped small, seasoned with Pepper and Salt, or, you may stuff it with Apples, or roast it without any Stuffing, but season it high, and roast it an Hour and a Quarter.

a Quarter. Put Gravy in the Dish, and Apple Sauce in a Bowl.

To roast Partridges.

AS they are roasting, baste them well and drudge them; put Gravy in the Dish under them, and make a Sauce thus: Boil some thin Slices of fine stale Bread, in as much Water as will make it thick and smooth, with whole Pepper, Mace, and an Onion stuffed with Cloves: When it is smooth, put in a good Piece of Butter; stir it and give it a Boil or two, put in a little Salt, so send it in a Sauce boat with your Partridges. You may lard them if you please.

To dress Partridges à la Braise.

TRUSS their Legs into their Bodies; give them a Scald, then lard them; season with Pepper, Salt, Cloves, and Mace, sweet Herbs, Chives, and Parsley, all shred, take a Stew-pan with a Cover, lay Slices of Bacon in it, then thin Slices of Beef over them, with Slices of Carots and Onions, Parsley, sweet Herbs, Pepper, Cloves, and Mace; then lay in the Partridges on their Breasts, and lay over them Slices of Beef, then Slices of Bacon; cover the Stew pan, and let them stew with Fire over and under them, make a Ragoo of Cocks Combs, Livers of fat Fowls, Sweet breads, Truffles, Mushrooms, Artichoke Bottoms, and Asparagus Tops, according to the Season, when your Partridges are stewed enough, take them up, drain them and dish them with the Ragoo about them, or, you may send them up with a Ragoo of Cucumbers, made thus: Pare and slice them, and some Shalots; put them between two Plates, with a little Pepper and Salt, for two Minutes; then drain off the Liquor that comes from them; then put them in a closs covered Pan with a Piece of Butter, and let them stew on a slow Fire till they are soft; then shake in a little Flour and Gravy, keeping them stirring all

all the while. Put in a chopped Anchovy, and a Spoonful of Ketchup.

Partridges with Oisters.

THEY must be very fresh, draw them; mince their Livers, and some scalded Oisters, the Yolks of hard Eggs, Parsley, sweet Herbs, and Shalots, shred small; Pepper, Salt, and Cloves, work them in a Piece of Butter, and stuff your Partridges with it; roll them up in Slices of Bacon, and Paper, spit them; then get some more Oisters, blanch and pick them; put them in some of their own Liquor, a little good Gravy, a Bit of Butter roll'd in Flour, a glass of white Wine, the Juice of half a Lemon with the Peel, Shalots cut small, pounded Mace, Pepper, and Salt; boil it, and dish your Partridges, and pour it round them.

To hash Partridges.

HALF roast your Partridges, cut them in Quarters, and joint the Breast and Rump asunder; put them in a Stew-pan, with some good Gravy, the Rind of a Lemon, an Onion stuffed with Cloves, Pepper, Salt, Mace, Truffles, and Morels; a Piece of Butter roll'd in Flour, a Glass of white Wine, and some Lemon Juice, let them all stew on the Fire a Quarter of an Hour, then dish them.

To roast Pheasants.

BLANCH and lard them with Bacon, then roll them in buttered Papers; roast them at a slow Fire: When almost done, take off the Papers to let them have a Colour, and dish them with good Gravy; send the same Bread-sauce as for Partridges, in a Sauce-boat with them. You may send either Oisters or Sellery Sauce with them.

To boil Pheasants, Partridges, Chickens, or Quails.

PUT them in a Stew-pan with as much Water as will cover them, with Mace, Nutmeg, Cloves, a Piece

N   of

of Butter, and some Crumbs of Bread; Lemon-peel,
Onions, and white Wine; let them all stew on a slow
Fire till enough; then take out the Lemon-peel and
Onion; turn your Fowl very often; put in the Yolks
of hard Eggs, chopped very fine, with a little more
Butter; give it a Boil, then dish them all up. Put in
the Juice of a Lemon.

A Pupton of Pigeons.

TAKE savoury Forc'd-meat rolled out like Paste,
in a butter'd Dish; lay Pigeons over it, then Sweet-
breads and Mushrooms, then another Roll of Forc'd-
meat; cover it and bake it: When enough, turn it on
another Dish, and your Gravy over it. Send it up hot.

Pigeons boiled with Rice.

STUFF their Bellies with chopped Parsley, Pepper and Salt rolled in a Bit of Butter, put them into
a Chopin of Broth, with a little beat Mace, a Bunch
of sweet Herbs, and an Onion; cover them close, and
let them stew for a Quarter of an Hour, then take
out the Onion and sweet Herbs, and take a good Piece
of Butter rolled in Flour, put it in and keep it stirring
till the Butter is dissolved, then have ready half a
Pound of Rice boiled tender, put it to the Pigeons,
with Salt and Nutmeg, give them a Scald, then put
the Pigeons in the Dish, and pour the Rice over them.

To stew Pigeons.

STUFF them with Forc'd meat, then half roast
them, then put them in a Stew-pan, with a Chopin
of Gravy, a little white Wine, or Claret, Pepper,
Cloves, Salt, Mace, Lemon-peel, pickled Mushrooms,
and Oisters, scalded and picked, with some of their
Liquor, and a scored Onion, let them stew till they
are done, thicken the Sauce with Butter and Flour,
take out the Onion, and send it up hot. You may do
Ducks the same Way.

To fry Pigeons.

BLANCH them and cut them in two, beat them flat, and put them in a Stew pan, with Onions, Parsley, Pepper, Salt, Cloves, a Piece of Butter, a Ladleful of Broth, or the Liquor they were in; let all these stew a little while, take them out and dip them in Batter made of Eggs and Flour, then fry them, dish them, and pour over them the Liquor they were stewed in, but strain it first: Put the Juice of a Lemon in it.

To broil Pigeons.

YOU may either broil them whole, or slit them down the Back, salt and pepper them, lay them on the Brander, broil them gently, and turn them often; make the Sauce of Butter, their Livers boiled and chopped with Parsley and Shalot: You may put a little red Wine in it, and Lemon Juice. If you do them whole, put Forc'd meat in them.

To boil Pigeons.

PUT them in warm Water to blanch, then boil them in Salt and Water fifteen Minutes; boil a Piece of Bacon, and take off the Skin, then put Crumbs of Bread on it, and lay it before the Fire, boil Spinage, Greens, or Colly-flowers, put the Bacon in the Dish, then the Pigeons, and the Garden Things about it. You may dress any tame Fowl the same Way: Don't put Salts in the Collyflowers when you boil them.

To do Pigeons à la Daube.

STUFF their Bellies with Forc'd meat made thus: Take a Pound of Veal, and a Pound of Beef Sewet, beat it in a Mortar, and season it with Pepper, Salt, and Nutmeg, put as much Crumbs of Bread as Sewet; brown them in clarified Butter, then shake in a little Flour, and put in it some good Gravy, and Onion stuffed with Cloves, Pepper, Salt, Mace, and Lemon-peel;

let

let them ſtew a while: Put a Ragoo of any Sort a-
bout them, or the Liquor they are ſtewed in.

Pigeons ſtoved with Cabbage Lettice.

STUFF them as before, ſeaſon them with Pepper, Salt, and Cloves, brown them with Butter, then
put them to ſtove with Cabbage Lettice cut in Quarters, and two green Onions, a little Gravy, a Glaſs of
Wine, and ſome Lemon Juice: Let them all ſtew on
a ſlow Fire, then diſh them. Put Forc'd-meat Balls
and Lemon about them.

Pigeons diſguiſed.

SEASON them with Pepper and Salt, make Puff
Paſte, and roll each Pigeon in Paſte; tye them in a
Cloth, boil them in a good deal of Water for an Hour,
untye them carefully that they don't break, diſh them
and pour Gravy about them. So ſerve them up hot.

A ſtewed Pheaſant.

STEW it in white Gravy, and when it is almoſt
enough, put in it Salt, Pepper and Mace, then take
boiled Artichoke Bottoms, Cheſnuts roaſted and ſkin-
ned, and put them in with a good Piece of Butter
rolled in Flour, a Glaſs of white Wine and Lemon
Juice: Let them ſtew a while, then diſh your Phea-
ſant and Sauce; put Forc'd-meat Balls or Sauſages a-
bout it: A good Fowl will do as well, but truſs it
with the Head on like a Pheaſant.

To roaſt Growſe, or what is called Moor-fowl.

TWO makes a Diſh; lard one of them, then ſpit
and roaſt them well; for the Sauce, take good brown
Gravy, Crumbs of Bread browned in a Pan, with a
very little Bit of Butter, a Gill of Claret, a ſhred Shal-
lot, Pepper and Salt.

To roast Snipes or Woodcocks.

DON'T draw them, slit them across, toast some Bread, and lay it in a Plate under them, that the Trale may drop in it: When roasted well, lay them on the toasted Bread, and pour beat Butter with Gravy over them: Send them up hot.

To stew Larks, or any other small Birds.

TOSS them in a Stew-pan with some Butter, an Onion stuck with Cloves, some Mushrooms, and the Livers of the Birds, with a little Gravy: Let them stew on a slow Fire; then beat two Eggs, with some shred Parsley; mix it by Degrees with the Sauce; put in some Salt and the Grate of a Lemon. Just as it is going to be dished, put in a little Lemon Juice.

To roast Larks.

PUT them on a Skewer, tye them to the Spit, baste them and drudge them with Crumbs of Bread and Salt; then have Crumbs of Bread, and lay it in the Dish with them.

To roast Curlews.

WHEN they are gutted, thrust them like a Woodcock, season them with Pepper and Salt: You may put Forc'd meat in them, roast them well, baste and drudge them, put Gravy, Claret and Orange Juice in the Dish under them.

To roast Quails.

STUFF their Bellies with Crumbs of Bread, chopped Parsley, Shalot, Oisters and sweet Marjoram; put a Piece of Butter in it, and a raw Egg, all work'd up together; then spit and roast them: When done, put Gravy, Anchovy, and the Juice of a Lemon in the Dish under them.

To

To roaſt Plovers.

PUT into their Bellies, Pepper, Salt, chopped Anchovies and Shalots: Don't roaſt them too much, and put good Gravy under them in the Diſh.

To ſtew Plovers.

SEASON them with Pepper, Salt and Cloves, put them in a Stew-pan with Gravy and Shalots; put them on a ſlow Fire; when they are half done, ſkim off all the Fat, and ſtrain it, then put into it two Gills of Claret, and an Onion ſtuffed with Cloves; then ſtove them till they are done; diſh them, and pour the Sauce over them. You may do wild Ducks, Teals or Widgeons the ſame Way. Take out the Onion.

A jugged Hare.

CUT it in Pieces, lard the Quarters with Bacon, put it in a Can that has a very narrow Mouth, with whole Pepper, Cloves and Mace: Cover the Can cloſs, that the Steam cannot come out; then put it in a Pot of Water, and let it boil in it three Hours, ſtill filling the Pot with Water up to the Can's Neck, but not as high as it can get into it. You may put Onions and a Faggot of ſweet Herbs in it, if you pleaſe; then put it in the Diſh, ſalt it to your Taſte, and take out the Herbs and Onions.

To roaſt a Hare.

LARD the Hare, and put a Stuffing in the Belly, with Crumbs of Bread, the Heart, Beef Sewet and the Liver chopped ſmall, Parſley, Onion and ſweet Herbs ſhred fine; ſeaſon it with Pepper, Salt, Nutmeg and the Grate of a Lemon; wet it with an Egg, then ſew it up and ſpit it, and baſte it with Cream till all the Blood is ſoak'd out: Let it dry, then flour and ſalt it, and baſte it with Butter: For Sauce, you may give it beat Butter, Gravy and Claret Sauce in a Boat.

To roaft a Hare another Way.

LARD the Hare, take grated Bread, Eggs, Currants, Nutmeg, Cinnamon, Sugar and a little Cream: Make all thefe in a Pudding, ftirring it in a Pan on the Fire for fix Minutes; then put it in the Hare's Belly, few it up, fpit it, roaft it, and bafte it with Butter. You may give it Claret Sauce and beat Butter.

To roaft a Hare with the Skin on.

TAKE out the Bowels, wipe the Infide with a Cloth, put a Pudding in it, of either favoury or fweet, as before; few the Belly up, then loofen all the Skin, and rub Butter all over the Flefh; then few up the Skin, and roaft it, bafting it with boiling Water and Salt, till it is half roafted, then let it dry; and when it fmokes, pull it off by Pieces, then bafte it with Butter, and drudge it with Flour or grated Bread. The Sauce is beat Butter, or Gravy and Claret.

To hafh a Hare.

HALF roaft it, then cut it in Quarters, put it in a Stew-pan, with Pepper, Salt, Cloves, Lemon-peel, whole Onions, a Bunch of fweet Herbs, and a little Gravy and Claret. You may thicken it a little with brown'd Butter and Flour: Take out the Lemon-peel, fweet Herbs and Onions.

To mince a Hare.

WHEN there is any Hare left that has been roafted, mince it fmall, put it in a Stew-pan, with two Gills of good Gravy, a little Parfley, Lemon-peel, Onions and fcalded Oifters all fhred fmall, a Piece of Butter rolled in Flour, Pepper, Salt and Mace, a Glafs of white Wine, and a little Lemon Juice: Give it two or three Boils, keeping it ftirring all the Time, then fend it up hot; or you may half roaft it, and then hafh it the fame Way.

To boil Rabbets.

LET them steep in warm Water a Quarter of an Hour, then put them in a Pot of boiling Water and Salt. Three Quarters of an Hour boils them. For the Sauce, you may boil Onions, chop them, and mix them with a Gill of Cream and a good Piece of Butter; pour it over them boiling hot, and put Salt in it; or you may boil the Livers, chop them with Parsley and Pickles, mix them with a Gill of Gravy, a good Piece of Butter rolled in Flour, and a little white Wine seasoned with Pepper, Salt, Mace and Nutmeg. You may lard them with Bacon if you like it.

Boiled Rabbets with Sausages.

STEW the Rabbets in as much Water as will cover them with Pepper, Salt, Cloves, Onions and sweet Herbs. When half done, take out the Rabbets, and strain the Broth, then blanch some Lettice and Spinage, and put them and the Rabbets in the Broth, with a Piece of Butter rolled in Flour, some Mushrooms or Truffles, if you have them: Fry Sausages, and when you dish the Rabbets and Sauce, put the Sausages about them. When you roast Rabbets, beat Butter, their own Liver, and Parsley minc'd small, is the Sauce.

To stew Rabbets the French Way.

CUT them in Quarters, lard them with Bacon, then stew them in strong Gravy, with a little white Wine, Pepper, Salt and Mace, browned Butter and Flour, and the Juice of a Lemon. Send them hot to Table.

To collar Salmon.

TAKE a Side of Salmon, cut a Piece of the Tail, rub the other Piece with Eggs, make a Forc'd-meat of the Tail, chop it small, with a Handful of Oisters that is parboiled, the Yolks of six Eggs boiled hard, and two Anchovies; chop them all small, season it with Pepper, Salt, Mace, Nutmeg, and some grated Bread, work

them

them up with two raw Eggs, and lay it all over the
Salmon, but firſt ſeaſon it with all the Spices as above.
Roll it up in a Collar, and bind it with broad Tape, and
boil it in boiling Water, Salt and Vinegar, for two Hours
on a ſlow Fire, then take it out and let it cool, and
ſkim all the Fat off the Water it was boiled in; take off
the Bindings of the Collar, and when both is cold, put
it in the Water it was boiled in.

To collar Pork.

TAKE a Piece of Pork and bone it, ſtrew it with
Salt, Pepper, Cloves, Mace, Parſley, Sage, Thyme
and ſweet Marjoram, all ſhred ſmall, then cut Slices
off a Leg of Veal, and ſeaſon them as above. Lay them
in the Pork, rub them and the Inſide of the Pork with
raw Eggs, then roll it up in a Collar very hard, bind
it with broad Tapes, and put it in a large Pot of boiling
Water. It will take three Hours boiling, then take it
out of the Pot, and when it is cold, you may make
Uſe of it, and keep it in the ſame Souſe you do Brawn.

To collar a Pig.

CUT off the Head and Feet, and ſlit it down the
Belly, take out all the Intrails, bone it, and lay it in
Water to ſoke out the Blood, then dry it with a Cloth,
ſeaſon it with chopped Sage and Parſley, white Pepper,
Salt and Mace, roll it up very hard, and roll a Cloth
about it; tye both Ends, put it in a Pot of boiling Wa-
ter, with a little Salt in it. It will, if large, take an
Hour and a half to boil it: When you take it out of
the Pot, hang it up by one End till it is almoſt cold:
You may ſend it to Table either whole or in Slices

To collar a Fore-quarter of Lamb, or a Breaſt of Veal.

BONE them and ſeaſon them with chopped Parſley and ſweet Herbs, black and *Jamaica* Pepper,
Cloves and Salt; roll them up hard, and bind them
with a Cloth tied at both Ends, put them in boiling

O Water.

Water. The Lamb will take an Hour and three Quarters, but the Veal will take but an Hour and a Half: Hang them by one End, till almoſt cold, then take them out of the Cloth.

To collar Cow Heels.

WHEN the Hair is well cleaned off the Feet, boil them till the Bones come out, then ſeaſon them with black and *Jamaica* Pepper, and Salt, roll them up tight, and boil them half an Hour more in their own Broth; hang them up till almoſt cold, then take them out of the Cloth.

To collar a Calf's Head.

CUT your Head in two, and waſh and ſoke it in warm Water, put it to boil, and when the Bones come out, ſeaſon it with Salt, Cloves, Pepper and Mace, then ſhread ſweet Marjoram, Thyme and Parſley, and ſtrew them on it, put the thin Part of one Side to the thick Part of the other, roll it up, and boil it for an Hour in its own Broth, then take it out, and hang it up till almoſt cold, then take it out of the Cloth.

To make a very good Collar of a Hog's Head.

WHEN it is clean waſhed, put it down to boil, and a Set of Cow Heels down with it; when boiled, take out all the Bones, and ſeaſon them with black and *Jamaica* Pepper and Salt, cut out the black of the Eye, put your Feet in the Middle, and roll it up very tight in a Cloth, boil it in its own Broth an Hour, hang it up by one End, and when almoſt cold, take it out of the Cloth. You may collar a Cow's Head the ſame Way, leaving out the Feet.

To collar Eels.

GET large Eels, cut off the Head and Fins, bone them, ſeaſon them with black and *Jamaica* Pepper, Cloves and Salt; roll them up very hard, and put them

down

down to boil in Water, Salt and Vinegar, with a few Bay Leaves: Boil them fo tender that you may thruft a Straw in them; take them out, and boil the Liquor better, with whole Spice in it. Let it cool, and fkim off all the Fat; then put in your Eels in your cold Liquor.

To pot a Cow's Head.

LET it blanch in Water all Night, then put it to boil, and when it is enough, all the Bones will come out; take out the black out of the Eyes, and cut it in thin Bits; feafon them with Pepper, Salt, Cloves and Mace, lay all the Bits in any Thing that will bear the Fire: You may have it in what Shape you pleafe, according to what you bake it in: Mind to put a Bit of Fat and Lean always together in different Pieces, one on the other; clarify a Chopin of the Broth it was boiled in, and when your Bits are all laid in your Can, pour it over them. You may put a Gill of white Wine and a Gill of Vinegar in it: Cover the Can clofe, and bake it two Hours. When it comes out of the Oven, put a light Weight on it, and when cold take it out. You may fend it to Table either whole or in Slices. It is to be eaten with Muftard, and Vinegar cold.

To pot Pigeons.

CUT off the Feet and Wings, feafon them with Salt and Pepper, chop the Liver and Gizzard very fmall, mix a good Handful of Crumbs of Bread with them, a little Parfley, Onion and Lemon-peel fhred fmall, a good Piece of Butter, wet it with an Egg, work it up together, and put it in the Pigeons Bellies; then put them in a Can with a good Piece of Butter; cover it clofe, and put it in the Oven: It is better than doing them on the Fire. You may do them without ftuffing if you pleafe. But you muft put Butter in their Bellies if you take them out of the Veffel that they were baked in, and put them in fmall Pots, they
will

will keep a long while; but you muſt drain all the Gravy from them, and put clarified Butter over them.

To make Liver Puddings.

HALF boil a Hog's Draught, mince it very ſmall; to every Pound of it, put a Pound of the Hog's Lard cut ſmall, or a Pound of Beef Sewet; you muſt put a Pound of Crumbs of Bread in it; ſeaſon it with Pepper, Salt and Clove Pepper: You may put Currants in them, if you pleaſe, wet it with a very little Water; fill and boil them as you do the Blood Puddings. If you put Currants in them, put a little Sugar too.

The proper Sauces for wild Fowl.

DUCKS, Veal and Plover muſt be roaſted very well; the Sauce is Gravy, Crumbs of Bread, Shalots, and a little Claret, ſeaſon it with Pepper and Salt. Partridges and Moor-fowl muſt be very well roaſted. Their Sauce is a little Bread boil'd in Water, a Blade of Mace, an Onion ſtuff'd with Cloves, a good Piece of Butter, and a little Salt: You may put a little white Wine and Ketchup in it. Woodcocks and Snipes are roaſted well, with their Guts in them; put toaſted Bread and beat Butter under them: Under other Fowls put Gravy; and put about any ſmall Birds fried Crumbs only. The proper Sauce for roaſted Veniſon is Claret boiled very thick, with Sugar or Currant Jelly.

To pot Woodcocks or Snipes.

DON'T take out the Traile, ſeaſon them with Salt and Clove Pepper, put them in a Can with a good deal of ſweet Butter, cover it cloſe, and bake them, when baked, take them out of the Can, and let all the Butter drain from them; put them in ſmall Pots, clarify the Butter they were in, add more to it, and pour it on them. Don't let any of the Gravy be in it. They muſt be covered with Butter.

To

To pot a Hare.

ROAST or bake the Hare, and when cold, pull all the Flesh from the Bones; pound it and season it with Pepper, Salt, Cloves, and Mace; put in an equal Quantity of sweet Butter as you have of Hare; clarify the Butter, and mix it with the Hare, then put it in small Pots; and when cold, pour clarified Butter on it: You may send it to Table in these Pots. You may pot Moor-fowl or Partridges the same Way.

To pot a Calf's Head.

BOIL it and two Calves Feet in as much Water as will cover them, with Pepper, Salt, Cloves, and Lemon-peel; boil it till the Bones come out, then strew on it a little Salt; boil the Broth it was boiled in till it is in a very stiff Jelly, cut the Head in thin Slices, the Breadth of a Crown; skin the Tongue and Palates, and slice them; cut the Eyes in round Rings; place them all regular in a Bowl that will bear the Oven; then take the Broth, and put in it whole Pepper, Cloves, Mace, and Lemon-peel, and the Juice of a Lemon, or a little Vinegar; clarify it with the Whites of two Eggs, and let it run through a Jelly-bag, then pour it over the Head, and put it in the Oven for half an Hour. The Oven must not be hot.

To pot Beef.

TAKE the Lean off a Buttock of Beef; cut some thin Pieces, and rub it with Salt-petre; let it lye in in it three Days, then dry it with a Cloth; put it in a flat Can, with Butter over and under it, cover the Can closs with coarse Paste; put it in the Oven for four Hours, then take it out and drain all the Butter and Gravy from the Beef; and when it is cold, and very clean of all the Fat, string it, and pound it very fine; rub it thro' a coarse Search, then season it with white Pepper, Cloves, Mace, and Salt; to every Pound of the Beef, after it is put through the Search, put a Pound

of

of clarified Butter, skim it clean, and pour it from the Bottom, that none of the Milk or Sediment go in it; then mix it with the Beef, and put it in small white Tart-pans; and when it is cold, pour clarified Butter over it. You may pot Venison the same Way.

To pot Tongues.

PICKLE them red, as you do to dry, then boil them tender, and peel them; rub them with Pepper, Cloves, and Mace; then turn them round on their Side in Pots that will hold but one, cover them with Butter; bake them when they come out of the Oven, pour off all the Gravy, and put the Butter that was over them, and more clarified Butter over them. They will keep a great while.

To pot Venison.

TAKE a Piece of Venison, Fat and Lean together, lay it in a Dish, and put Pieces of Butter over it; tye over the Dish some coarse Paper or brown Dough, put it in the Oven, and bake it very well, then take it out of the Gravy, and when it is cold and well drain-ed, pound it, both Fat and Lean, but first skin and bone it, season it with Salt, Pepper, Cloves, Nutmeg and Mace, all pounded fine, then clarify the Butter that it was baked in, with as much added to it as will moisten it, and put it in small potting Pots. You must be sure to take out all the Strings, and let it be beat to a Paste. Cover the Pots with clarified Butter.

To pot Beef or Venison in Slices.

TAKE lean Beef, and cut it in Slices, beat them with the Roller, and lard them; season them with Pepper, Salt, Cloves and Mace, put them in a Dish, and bake them with Butter over them; cover them close. You may put Onions and sweet Herbs to them, if you please. They are to be eaten either hot or cold.

To pot Salmon the Newcastle *Way.*

TAKE the Salmon, and scale and wipe it very clean, but don't wash it; salt it well, then let it lye till the Salt is melted and drained from it, then season it with Pepper, Cloves and Mace: Put it in a Pot with Butter over it, cover it closs, and bake it: When baked, pour all the Gravy from it; and when it is cold, put clarified Butter over it. You may do Carp, Tench, Trouts, and several Kinds of Fish, the same Way.

To pot a *Pike.*

SCALE it, and cut off the Head, split it, take out the Bones, wipe it clean, and salt the Inside with Bay Salt and Pepper; roll it up round, and put it in a Pot with Butter over it, cover it closs, bake it an Hour, then pour all the Liquor from it, and lay it to drain on a Cloth, then put it in a potting Pot, and pour clarified Butter on it.

To make Marrow *Pasties.*

CUT half a Pound of Marrow in Bits, shread six Apples, and the Yolks of three hard Eggs, a Pound of Currants, pick them clean, plump them before the Fire, and mix all together; season it with the Grate of a Lemon, pounded Cinnamon, Mace, Nutmeg, a very little Sugar and Salt: Put them in Puff Paste. You may either bake or fry them.

To dress a Veal or Lamb's Ear, *properly called* Kidneys.

SLIT the Kidneys, Fat and all, rub it with an Egg, strew on it Crumbs of Bread, Parsley, Thyme, Onion, Pepper and Salt; fry it in a Pan. You may mince it if you please, and season it with Sugar, Nutmeg, and a little Salt; wash a few Currants in warm Water, and plump them before the Fire: Mix all together with the Grate of a Lemon, roll a little Puff Paste, and fry them in it. You may make them without Sugar or

Currants,

Currants, if you pleafe ; and if you put an Egg in them, you may do them on Toafts before the Fire.

To make Blood Puddings.

WHEN the Beaft is killing, ftir the Blood with your Hand, and break the Lumps : Put Salt in it, while hot, ftrain it, boil a Chopin of Groats in Milk, and put them in when they both are cold. To every Pint of this, put a Pound of chopped Sewet, fhred fweet Herbs and Onions ; feafon it to your Tafte with Pepper and Salt, clean the Skins very well, fill three Parts of them, tye them, have a Pot of boiling Water, and put them in : Let them not boil at firft, but take them out and prick them a little to let out the Wind : When they are almoft cold, put them in again. Do this three or four Times, till they are a little hard, then they won't burft in the boiling ; ftir them in the Skins when you are putting them firft down.

To make a Yorkſhire Pudding.

BEAT eight Eggs, and beat in them a Pound of Flour, putting a Mutchkin of Milk in by Degrees in it, fhread half a Pound of Beef Sewet very fine, and mix in it ; feafon it with Salt and Ginger, three Hours boils it. You may bake a Pudding made the fame Way.

To make a Plumb Pudding.

BEAT eight Eggs and half a Pound of Flour, two Gills of Milk, and half a Pound of Raifins fhred, half a Pound of Currants wafhed and picked clean, half a Pound of Beef Sewet fhred fmall, and mix all toge ther ; feafon it with Nutmeg, Ginger, Salt, and a Glafs of Brandy. Two Hours boils it.

To make Almond Puddings in Lemon or Orange Skins.

BOIL your Skins, firft cut a Hole on the Top, and take out all the Infide, boil them tender in Wa- ter, then boil them in Syrup, blanch a Quarter of a

                                                    Pound

Pound of sweet Almonds, and four bitter ones, pound them fine, mix them with a Gill of Cream, two Eggs, and two Spunge Biscuits; crumb them small; season it with Sugar to your Taste, put them in a Sauce-pan, and stir them one Way on the Fire, till the Rawness is off the Eggs: Take care it does not curdle; then fill your Skins, and put the Bit that you cut out in its Place again. This is enough for an Ashet. Send them hot to the Table.

To make a Pease Pudding.

TAKE a Pound of split Pease, and tye them in a Cloth, giving them Room to swell. Let them boil an Hour, then take them up, and blend them with a Spoon, put in them a good Piece of Butter, a little Salt and Pepper. Put them again in the Pot, let them boil half an Hour, and put beat Butter about them.

To make an Almond Pudding.

BLANCH and pound half a Pound of sweet Almonds, and six bitter ones, very fine, keeping them wetting as they are pounding with Brandy or Ratafia; beat the Yolks of twelve Eggs to a Cream, and pound and sift half a Pound of Sugar, and mix it with your Eggs by Degrees, keeping them whisking all the Time; then your Almonds, then put in six Ounces of oiled Butter, put it in the Oven as soon as you can, with Puff Paste about the Dish. You may make half the Quantity of any of these Puddings, if you please to try them, but put them in a very small Ashet. They are all approved Receipts.

To make a Citron Pudding.

POUND five Ounces of Citron very fine, with six Ounces of fine Sugar: Beat the Yolks of nine Eggs to a Cream, and whisk them together, with a Spoonful of the Juice of Spinage, and a little Brandy. Just as it is going into the Oven, put into it six Onnces of

P   oiled

oiled Butter   Half an Hour bakes it.   Keep it beating till it goes into the Oven.

To make a Rice Pudding.

WASH your Rice very well, and boil half a Pound in a Chopin of new Milk, till it is almoſt dry, then ſtir ſix Ounces of Butter in it, and let it cool a little, beat five Eggs, but three of the Whites, mix all together with a Gill of Cream, the Grate of an Orange or Lemon, a Quarter of a Pound of powdered Sugar, and a little Brandy. You may put Currants or Raiſins in it, if you pleaſe.   Put Paſte about the Diſh, put a little beat Cinnamon and Nutmeg in it.

Another Way to make a Rice Pudding.

BOIL a Chopin of Milk, and thicken it with four large Spoonfuls of the Flour of Rice, blend the Rice in a little cold Cream or Milk, then ſtir it in your Milk on the Fire, with grated Lemon-peel and Nutmeg, ſweeten it to your Taſte, and when boiled pretty thick, take it off, and ſtir in it five Ounces of Butter, ſet it to cool, beat ſix Eggs, but three Whites, and when it is cold, mix them together, and put Paſte about the Diſh.   You may make an Oat-meal Pudding the ſame Way.   Put a little beat Cinnamon in them, and Nutmeg.

To make a Potatoe Pudding.

BOIL the large white Potatoes, peal and pound half a Pound of them very well, beat twelve Eggs, four Whites, very thick, and whiſk in them half a Pound of fine powdered Sugar, then your Potatoes, grated Nutmeg, and a large Glaſs of Brandy. Put half a Pound of oiled Butter in it.   Juſt as it is going into the Oven, put Puff Paſte about the Diſh. It takes three Quarters of an Hour to bake it.   You may make a Carot Pudding the ſame Way.

T

To make a Sagoe Pudding.

WASH and pick your Sagoe, put it to boil in a Chopin of Water : There muſt be half a Pound of Sagoe, boil it with the Rind of a Lemon, and a Stick of Cinnamon ; when boiled pretty ſtiff, put in two Gills of white Wine, and a grated Nutmeg : Take it up, and when cold, put to it ſix Eggs, but three Whites, well beaten ; ſweeten it to your Taſte, and put it in the Oven, not too hot : When the Paſte is baked, it is enough. You may make a Millet Pudding the ſame Way, but there muſt be eight Eggs, and half the Whites in it.

To make an Apple Pudding.

BAKE or roaſt ſix or ſeven large Apples, ſkin and core them, then rub them through a Search with the Back of a Spoon, beat a Quarter of a Pound of Biſcuit, and mix with it, then beat eight Eggs, but three Whites, and beat them all up very well together, with beat Cinnamon, the Grate of a Lemon, and a little Orange-flower Water ; ſweeten it to your Taſte, and juſt as you are going to put it in the Oven, put into it four Ounces of clarified Butter. Put Puff Paſte about it   A little bakes it.

To make a Gooſe-berry Pudding.

SCALD two Chopins of Gooſe-berries, and rub them through a Search with the Back of a Spoon : Pound ſix Ounces of Spunge Biſcuits, and mix with them eight Eggs, but half the Whites, and half a Pound of fine powdered Sugar ; then put in the reſt with Orange-flower Water. A very little bakes it.

To make a Tanſy Pudding.

BEAT ten Eggs, with eight Ounces of fine Sugar, then put in half a Mutchkin of Spinage Juice, a Mutchkin of Cream, a little Brandy and Nutmeg, eight Ounces of Spunge Biſcuit, or white Bread grated fine, a little Juice of Tanſy to your Taſte, the Tanſy muſt be pounded and ſhred , a Quarter of a Pound of blanched and
pounded

pounded Almonds; mix all thefe well together in a Stew-pan, with three Ounces of Butter; fet it on the Fire, ftirring it till it is hard, then put it in your Difh, and bake it. Strew Sugar and fliced Orange on it. You may make a Tanfy without Almonds the fame Way.

To make a Marrow Pudding.

LAY thin Slices of Bread on your Difh, then lay on your Marrow in Lumps, then ftrew on Currants, fo fill your Difh or Pudding pan with Lairs; put a little beat Cinnamon, Nutmeg and Mace between the Lairs; beat eight Eggs, but two Whites, and a Chopin of Milk fweetened to your Tafte; cover it. You may bake it without a Cover, if you pleafe.

To make an Oat-meal Pudding.

BOIL a Quart of Water, feafon it with Sugar, Salt, Brandy and Nutmeg; thicken it with Oat-meal till you can hardly ftir the Spoon in it, add to it half a Pound of Currants, butter your Pan very thick. Pour it in, and half an Hour bakes it.

To make a Four-hour Pudding.

STONE and mince a Pound of Raifins, wafh and pick a Pound of Currants, mince a Pound of Beef Sewet very fine; beat eight Eggs with four Spoonfuls of Flour, a Gill of Brandy, a little Bit of Cinnamon, and Nutmeg, ftir them all together, butter your Bag, and tye it up very clofs; leave no Room, for it will not fwell: You muft boil it four Hours. The Sauce is Butter and Wine.

To make a Bread Pudding.

CUT all the foft of a Penny Loaf; boil a Mutch-kin of Milk with a Stick of Cinnamon, and the Rind of a Lemon, and pour it on your Bread, your Bread muft be cut in thin Slices; cover it up clofs for half an Hour; beat fix Eggs, a little Sugar, a Glafs of Brandy
and

and Nutmeg; mix all with your Bread: You may put in Currants, and a little Beef Sewet, if you pleafe; butter your Bag, and tye it up very clofs; an Hour and an half boils it; an Hour, if there is not Sewet and Currants in it.

To make a Flour Pudding.

BEAT eight Eggs, and mix in it three Spoonfuls of Flour, the Grate of a Lemon, Nutmeg, Sugar, a Glafs of Brandy, a little Salt and a Mutchkin of Milk, butter and flour your Cloth; tye it up clofs, it takes three Quarters of an Hour to boil; let it, and all Puddings that are boiled, be put in boiling Water, and the Boil never given over till you fend them up: Melted Butter and Wine is the beft Sauce for thefe Puddings. Keep them ftirring in the Pot as they are boiling.

A boiled Rice Pudding.

TAKE half a Pound of Rice, tye it loofe in a Cloth, and boil it half an Hour; then add to it a good Piece of Butter, a little Cinnamon, Sugar, Salt and the Grate of a Lemon, ftir all together and tye it up very clofs; then boil it for an Hour. White Wine and Butter is the Sauce.

To make a Sewet Pudding.

SHREAD a Pound of Sewet very fine, a Pound of Flour, a Pound of Currants, fix Eggs, a little Ginger, Nutmeg, Sugar and Brandy; mix all together. Boil it three Hours.

To make an Oat-meal Pudding.

GET a Mutchkin of coarfe Oat-meal, a Pound of Sewet fhred fmall, half a Pound of Currants; feafon it with Sugar, Salt, Nutmeg, Mace and the Grate of a Lemon; beat four Eggs and add to it; put it in your Cloth, and leave Room for it to fwell. Two Hours will boil it.

To

To make a Custard Pudding.

BOIL a Mutchkin of Cream, with a Stick of Cinnamon, and the Rind of a Lemon and Orange; sweeten it to your Taste; beat the Yolks of eight Eggs, and mix your Cream in them by Degrees, butter a white Stone Bowl, and put it in it; then butter a thick Piece of Cloth, and tye it on the Bottom of the Bowl; turn the Top down in boiling Water half an Hour, boil it, and tye it very fast.

An Orange Custard, or Pudding.

RUB the Outside of four *Seville* Oranges with Salt, then pare them; lay the Peel in Water till the Bitterness is off them; then pound them very fine, and put in the Yolks of ten Eggs, and a Chopin of Cream, mix them well, and sweeten them to your Taste, put half a Pound of clarified Butter in it, if you bake it for a Pudding, and Puff Paste about the Dish; but if for Custards, put no Butter in, but put it in Cups. They both are to be baken.

To make a Lemon Pudding.

GRATE the Rind of three clear Lemons, put it to steep in Brandy; then grate two *Naples*, or Spunge Biscuits, and mix with it, beat the Yolks of ten Eggs and two of the Whites, and pound eight Ounces of Sugar very fine, and with the Eggs put in the Biscuits, the Rind of the Lemon and Brandy, keeping it beating all the while; put Puff Paste about the Dish, and just as you are going to put it in the Dish, beat in half a Pound of clarified Butter. The Butter must be almost cold.

A Carot Pudding.

BOIL as many good Carots as will be half a Pound, cut them and pound them fine with half a Pound of fine Sugar; then beat ten Eggs and three Whites, and mix them with the Carots, grate an Orange in it, and just as you are going to put it into the

Oven,

Oven, put into it half a Pound of clarified Butter. All the Butter that is put in baked Puddings muſt be clarified, and the Skin and Bottom taken from it.

A Yellow Pudding.

GRATE the Crumbs of a fine Two-penny Loaf, and put it in a Pudding Diſh, and pour on it three Mutchkins of Milk or Cream, five or ſix Eggs, a Pound of Beef Sewet, half a Pound of Raiſins, and a Pound of Currants, ſome Saffron ſteeped in Roſe Water, and ſtrained into it; ſweeten it to your Taſte, and bake it. Pour the Milk on the Bread boiling hot.

To make a Barley Pudding.

PUT to a Quart of Cream or Milk, the Yolks of ſix Eggs and three Whites, beat them well; ſeaſon it with Nutmeg, Salt, a little Orange-flower Water, and the Grate of an Orange and Lemon; then put in ſix Handfuls of Pearl Barley, but boil it a little in Milk firſt; put in it twelve Ounces of melted Butter, mix all together, with ſix Ounces of Sugar; butter a Diſh, and pour it in. It takes a good while to bake it.

To make a boiled Apple Pudding.

MAKE a good Puff Paſte, roll it out half an Inch thick, pare the Apples and ſcore them; fill the Paſte and cloſe it up, tye it in a Cloth, and boil it two Hours, if a large one three, then turn it out into the Diſh; cut a Piece out of the Top of the Paſte, and put Butter and Sugar in it to your Taſte; then lay on the Piece again. A Pear, Damſons, or any Sort of Plumbs, Apricock, Cherries, Raſpberries, Currants, Gooſe-berries, or Mulberry Puddings may be made the ſame Way. Send beat Butter, a little white Wine and Sugar in a Bowl.

To make an Orange Pudding.

BOIL the Skins of three Oranges very tender
pound them very fine in a marble or wooden Mortar,
pound half a Pound of fine Sugar, and beat the Yolks
of twelve Eggs to a Cream; mix your Sugar in them,
then your Orange, beat them very well together,
have eight Ounces of Butter melted to Oil, skim and
bottom it; let it be as cold, that it will but just
pour before you put it in, and don't put it in till you
are putting the Pudding in the Oven; put Puff Paste
about the Dish, wipe it up before you put it in the
Dish; half an Hour bakes it. You must oil, skim and
bottom all your Butter for baked Puddings, and let
it be almost cold before you put it in.

To make a Lemon Pudding.

GRATE the Rind of four Lemons, and put it in
a Glass of Brandy; beat the Yolks of ten Eggs, till
they are very thick, and pound and sift half a Pound
of Sugar, and beat it up well with your Eggs, then
put in the Lemon Rind, and just as it is going into
the Oven, put in eight Ounces of Butter, as above,
put Puff Paste about the Dish of all baked Puddings
Half an Hour bakes it. Boil two Lemon Skins, and
pound and mix them with this.

To make a Pudding of whole Rice.

PUT half a Pound of cold Butter on the Bottom
of your Pudding pan; strew over it six Ounces of
Rice, then half a Pound of Raisins or Currants, a
grated Nutmeg; put over it two Chopins of new
Milk: You may colour it with Saffron, it both eats
and looks the better; grate the Rind of a Lemon, or
Orange in it, don't stir it, but put it in a very hot
Oven: It takes two Hours to bake it, sweeten it
to your Taste, always stone the Raisins, wash, dry
and pick the Currants, and wash and dry your Rice.

To

To make Clary-Cake.

BEAT fix Eggs very well with Salt and Nutmeg; fhread a Handful of Clary, and mix with them; fry them, or put it in a Difh in the Driping pan when Meat is roafting, and it will bake. You may make one the fame Way with Chives and Parfley.

To make Pancakes.

BEAT fix Eggs, and thicken them well with Flour, a little Ginger and Nutmeg, a little Salt, Sugar, and a Glafs of Brandy; put to them a Mutchkin of Milk; fry them in Butter, either thick or thin, as you like.

To make Cuftard Pancakes

BEAT eight Eggs; mix in them, with four Spoonfuls of Flour, a Glafs of Brandy, a little Ginger and Nutmeg, Sugar, and the Grate of a Lemon; put to them a Mutchkin of Cream, and a little melted Butter; they will not turn in the Pan, but you muft hold the upper Side to the Fire till crifp.

To make Pancakes.

BEAT four Eggs, a little Ginger, Nutmeg, and Salt; make them thick with Flour, then put in a Mutchkin of Two-penny, fry them crifp, and then you may put in Sugar, if you pleafe.

To make Apple Dumplins.

MAKE Puff Pafte, not too rich, and pare and fcoop out the Cores of as many large Apples as will fill your Difh at the black End, then put in the Place where you fcoop out the Core, Currant-jelly, or Marmalade of Oranges, roll out your Pafte thin, and roll up the Apples in it feparately, tye them up in Pieces of Cloth, and put them in a Pot of boiling Water: An Hour and a half boils them. Melted Butter, white Wine, and Sugar, is the proper Sauce.

To

To make fried Pan Puddings.

TO a Mutchkin of Milk put three Quarters of a Pound of Flour, fix Ounces of Beef Sewet fhred as fine as Flour, fix Ounces of Currants wafhed and plumped, a little Salt, Nutmeg, a Glafs of Brandy, and three or four Eggs, mix all well together; fry them in a Pan of Fat, and make them a little larger than Fritters.

Pancakes.

TAKE five Eggs, beat them very well with fix Spoonfuls of Flour, the Grate of a Lemon, a little Ginger and Salt, and a Mutchkin of Milk, fry them very crifp, and then ftrew Sugar on them, and fend them in very hot.

To make French Fritters.

TAKE two Gills of Water, an Ounce of Butter, a little Cinnamon, Sugar and Brandy, and grated Lemon-peel; fet it over the Fire, and boil the Water, ftir in the Flour as faft as you can, till in a Pafte, work it till it is like Pafte for ten Minutes; put it in a Bowl, work it with the Yolks of fix Eggs and one White, till it is in a light Pafte, drop them in a Pan of boiling Fat, with a Spoon or a Knife; fry them a light brown, diffi them, and throw Sugar on them.

To make Apple Fritters.

BEAT four Eggs, make them pretty thick with Flour, put two Gills of Milk, a little Salt, Sugar, and Nutmeg into it; it muft be as thick that it will ftick to the Apples, pare and cut them in thin Slices, and take out the Cores, but don't break the Slices, put them in the Batter, and have a good deal of boiling Beef-driping, and drop them in one by one till your Pan is full, fry them a light brown, then take them out, and put in more till they are all done, ftrew on them Sugar when you difh them: Any Kitchen-
fee

fee that is fweet and clean will fry them. All Fritters are fried the fame Way.

To make Potatoe Fritters.

BOIL and pound fix Potatoes, mix them with five Eggs well beaten, a Gill of Cream, a little Sugar, Nutmeg, the Grate of an Orange, two Ounces of oiled Butter, and a little Brandy; beat all well together, drop them in a Pan almoft full of boiling Fat, and fry them a light brown. Strew Sugar on them when difhed.

To make Currant Fritters.

BEAT four Eggs with fix Spoonfuls of Flour, and a little Salt, Sugar, Nutmeg, Ginger, and the Grate of a Lemon, then put in it half a Mutchkin of Cream, a Dram, and a Quarter of a Pound of Currants wafhed, picked and dried, drop them by Spoonfuls in a Pan almoft full of boiling Fat. Fry them a light brown.

To make Barm Dumplins.

MAKE a light Dough, as for Bread, with Barm, Flour, an Egg and Water, then boil a Panful of Water, and put the Dough in it, making it into little round Balls as big as an Egg, then flat them with your Hand, and put them in the boiling Water: Ten Minutes boils them Take Care they don't fall to the Bottom. Send them to the Table with beat Butter in a Cup. Put Salt in them.

To make Hard Dumplins.

MIX Flour and Water, an Egg, and a little Salt, like a Pafte, roll them as before, then boil them in boiling Water for half an Hour · They are beft boiled with Beef. Send Butter in a Cup with them.

Another Way to make Apple Dumplins.

PARE and core your Apples, and cut them in fmall Pieces, then pare and core a Quince, and grate it among the Apples, then make a good Puff Pafte; roll

it in small Pieces, and put in the Apples and Quinces;
fasten them up and tye them in different Places in a
Cloth, and boil them, and when they are enough,
take them out of the Cloth, cut a Bit out of the Top,
and put in them Sugar and Butter, then dish them,
and put the Tops on them again.

A Florendine of Oranges, or Apples.

CUT half a Dozen *Seville* Oranges into Slices, and
save the Juice· take out the Pulp, and lay them in
Water twelve Hours, then boil them in Water till they
are tender, keeping the Pan full of Water all the
Time, then boil all the·Juice, with a Pound of Sugar, and the Oranges cut in thin Slices, then boil ten
Pipins in Water and Sugar, put them in the Dish, and
half the Oranges among them; cover it with a Lid of
carved Puff Paste. A Florendine of Currants is made
the same Way.

An Almond Florendine.

BLANCH and beat very fine a Pound of Almonds
with Orange flower Water, beat eight Eggs, but half
of the Whites, mix them with two Gills of Cream,
and half a Gill of Brandy, half a Pound of clarified
-Butter, a Pound of Currants well washed and picked,
season it with Sugar, Cinnamon, and Nutmeg, all pound
ed fine; mix them all very well, put them in a Dish
with Puff Paste under and over them: You may put
candied Lemon, and Citron in thin Slices in it, if you
please. A little while bakes it.

To make a plain Tansy.

TAKE a fine stale Penny Loaf, and cut the Crumb
in thin Shaves; put it in a Bowl, then boil a Mutchkin
of Cream, and when boiled, pour it over the Bread, then
cover the Bowl with a Plate, and let it ly a Quarter of an
Hour; then mix it with eight Eggs well beaten, two
Gills of the Juice of Spinage, two Spoonfuls of the
Juice of Tansy, and sweeten it with Sugar, Nutmeg,
and

and a little Brandy; rub your Pan with Butter, and put it in it; then keep it ſtirring on the Fire till it is pretty thick, then put it in a buttered Diſh; you may either bake it, or do it in the Driping-pan under roaſted Meat.

To boil a Tanſy.

CUT the Bread, as in the other Tanſy, and pour a Mutchkin of boiling Milk on it, cover it up, then beat eight Eggs with a little of the Grate of a Lemon, or Orange, Nutmeg and Sugar; put to it ſome Juice of Spinage, and a little Tanſy Juice; ſtir all well together, then tye it up in a Cloth, and boil it an Hour and an Half; when you diſh it, ſtick it with candied Orange, and cut a *Seville* Orange in Quarters round it; ſend beat Butter, white Wine and Sugar in a Cup with it to the Table.

A Pipin Tanſy.

PARE and cut as many Pipins as will cover the Bottom of a Diſh, then take half a Penny Loaf, crumb it fine, pour on it a Mutchkin of Cream, and eight Eggs well beaten, ſeaſon it with Sugar, Nutmeg and Ginger, put in a Gill of Spinage Juice, and a Spoonful of Tanſy Juice, beat all together, then put in your Slices of Apples, butter your Frying-pan, and put in the Tanſy; when the Pan is hot, you muſt fry it on both Sides, or you may bake it in the Oven; ſend beat Butter, Orange and Sugar to Table with it.

To make a white Pot.

TAKE two Chopins of Milk, mix with it nine Eggs well beaten, a little Roſe Water, grated Lemon-peel, Nutmeg and Sugar, cut the Crumb of a Penny Loaf n thin Slices, and lay them in a Pudding-pan, then pour the Milk over them. You muſt put a little Butter on the Top. Put it in a ſlow Oven. Half an Hour bakes it.

Another

Another Sort of White Pot.

LAY a Lair of Marrow on the Bottom of the Dish you intend to bake it in, then lay all over it Slices of fine Bread cut very thin, strew over the Bread ston'd Raisins, putting grated Lemon-peel, Nutmeg and Ginger between them; then take a Chopin of Cream, and seven or eight Eggs well beaten with Sugar and a little Nutmeg; mix them with the Cream, and pour it over them softly, till the Dish is full: Let it stand a while before you put it in the Oven: Lay Slices of Bread, and Bits of Butter on the Top of all. You may make it with Currants, if you please.

A Rice White Pot.

BOIL a Chopin of Cream or Milk, then put in two Ounces of pick'd Rice, Sugar, Ginger, Cinnamon and Mace beaten, set it by to cool, beat six Yolks of Eggs, and two Whites, and mix them with the Cream, then put in four Ounces of pick'd and washed Currants, and a little Salt. You may bake it with or without Paste, boil the Rice a little, or put the Powder of Rice in it, instead of whole Rice.

Pancakes Royal.

MIX two Gills of Cream with two Gills of Sack, then beat up twelve Eggs, with Sugar, Cinnamon, Nutmeg and Ginger; mix them with as much Flour as will let them turn, then put in the Cream, and fry them with clarified Butter. The Pan must be always hot before you fry Pancakes.

Common Pancakes.

TAKE a Chopin of Milk, eight Spoonfuls of Flour, grated Nutmeg and Ginger, beat all together with a Glass of Brandy, let it stand a while, then fry them, and send them in hot with Sugar and Oranges,

Irish *Pancakes.*

BOIL a Mutchkin of Cream, with the Rind of an Orange, and some Cinnamon, then set it to cool: Beat eight Eggs, and but four of the Whites, with Sugar, Nutmeg, a little Salt, and two Gills of Flour; then beat three Ounces of sweet Butter, and mix the Cream and Eggs together, with a Glass of Brandy: Put a very little Bit of Butter in the Frying-pan, and when it is hot, put in two Gills of the Batter: They will not turn, but you must hold them before the Fire, to brown the upper Side.

To make Rice Pancakes.

BOIL a Chopin of Cream, thicken it with three Spoonfuls of the Flour of Rice, stir in half a Pound of Butter, and a grated Nutmeg: put it to cool, then beat eight Eggs, and mix with the Cream, put in a little Salt, and sweeten it to your Taste; mix them well, and fry them in Butter; serve them up hot; if they don't fry well, put in a Spoonful of Flour.

Oat-meal Pancakes.

BOIL a Chopin of Milk, and blend in it a Mutchkin of the Flour of Oat-meal thus: Keep a little Milk, and mix the Meal by Degrees in it, then stir in the boiling Milk, when it is pretty thick, put it to cool, then beat up six Eggs with Sugar, Nutmeg, the Grate of a Lemon and a little Salt: Stir all together, and fry them in Butter, putting in a Spoonful of the Batter at a Time. Serve them up hot, with beat Butter, Orange and Sugar.

Chopped Apples in small Pancakes.

TAKE a Mutchkin of Milk, sweeten it to your Taste, then beat six Eggs, with Nutmeg and the Grate of Lemon peel; mix them with five or six Spoonfuls of Flour, then put in the Milk by Degrees, a Glass of Brandy, a little Salt and Ginger; beat them up well,

then

then put in chopped Apples. It muft be pretty thick with them, then fry them in fmall Pancakes.

To make crifp Pancakes.

TAKE four Eggs with Ginger and Salt, mix in them fix or feven Spoonfuls of Flour, and a Mutchken of Two-penny. You may put Lemon-peel and Nutmeg in them; fry them very thin in Butter · When you fry them firft, if there is not enough of Flour, put in a little more.

To make a Clary Amulet.

BEAT eight or ten Eggs, with a little Pepper, Salt and Nutmeg; then put into it two Gills of Cream, and a Handful of Clary chopped very fine: Mix them well together, put fome Butter or Beef-dripings in your Frying pan, and when it is boiling hot, pour in your Amulet; fry it on both Sides, and fend it up hot. You may make one of Parfley and Chives the fame Way.

To poach Eggs and Spinage.

BOIL the Spinage in Water and Salt; chop them very fmall, then fqueeze them between two Trenchers, and mix them with a good Piece of fweet Butter, falt them to your Tafte, then poach fix or feven Eggs in boiling Water and Salt, letting the Water boil before you break in the Eggs, place the Spinage in an Afhet, then lay the Eggs over them; take them up with an Egg-fpoon, and don't break them, poach Eggs for Gravy the fame Way; pour the Gravy fcalding hot in the Difh, and lay your poache'd Eggs in it.

Eggs with Cabbage Lettice.

SCALD fome Cabbage Lettice in Water; fqueeze them well, then flice them and tofs them up in Butter, with a little Gravy; feafon it with Pepper and Salt, then let them ftew for half an Hour on a flow Fire, being clofs covered; then poach Eggs, and lay over them

them when they are difhed : You may put Saufages in the Difh round them.

To butter Eggs.

TAKE eight Eggs ; put them in a Stew-pan after they are well beaten with a little Salt and Nutmeg ; put to them a Quarter of a Pound of fweet Butter, and a Spoonful of fweet Cream, keep them ftirring all the Time they are on the Fire from the Bottom of the Pan, then put them on toafted Bread when they are thick.

Fried Bacon and Eggs.

CUT thin Slices of Bacon, and fry them a light brown ; then take them up and clean the Pan, cover them, put a little Butter in the Pan, when it is clarified, break into it your Eggs ; when they are a light brown, hold the Pan before the Fire to harden the other Side, for they muft not be turned : Put the Bacon in the Difh, and the Eggs over them.

To make an Amulet.

GET what Quantity of Eggs you think will fill the Difh ; feafon them with Pepper and Salt ; ten Eggs will fill a fmall Difh ; fhread Parfley and Chives, and beat them and the Eggs with a Gill of Cream very well ; then fry them in a Pan of good clarified Butter or Beef-driping on both Sides . You may put in Gravy inftead of Cream : You may put cut Slices of Oranges over it in the Difh.

Eggs and the Juice of Sorrel.

POACH your Eggs in Water, and have fome Sorrel pounded ; put the Juice of it in a Difh with fome Butter, two or three raw Eggs, and Salt and Nutmeg ; make all in a Sauce, and pour it on your poached Eggs. So ferve them up.

R   *A*

A pretty Dish of Whites of Eggs.

TAKE the Whtes of twelve Eggs, beat them up with four Spoonfuls of Rose Water, a little grated Lemon-peel, Nutmeg and Sugar, mix them well, and boil them in four small Bladders; tye them in the Shape of an Egg, and boil them hard, they will take half an Hour; lay them in the Dish, when they are cold mix two Gills of Cream with half a Gill of Malaga, a little Orange juice and Sugar; then take out the Eggs, and pour the Cream over them in the Dish.

Eggs poached in Cream.

FILL a Dish almost full of Cream; put it on the Fire, and when the Cream boils, break as many Eggs in it as the Dish will hold; season it with Pepper, Salt, and Nutmeg; cover them with another Dish, but take care they are not too hard. Then serve them up.

Oisters or Cockles fried with Eggs.

WASH them well in their own Liquor; give them a Scald, let them cool; then beat ten or twelve Eggs, and mix them with Crumbs of Bread, Pepper, Nutmeg, and Salt, put in a Gill of Cream, beat them well, then put in your Oisters or Cockles; have the Pan with clarified Butter, then drop them in; turn them, and fry them a light brown · When one Panful is done, put more, so do till they are done. You may send Butter and Lemon juice in a Cup, or Gravy. They are very pretty to garnish any Dish of Fish

To make Puff Paste.

TO two Pound of Flour, you must have a Pound of Butter; rub in the Flour two Ounces of the Butter, and put in it two Eggs; then wet it cold, wet as much as will make a stiff Paste; work it very smooth, then roll out the Paste, and stick it all over with Butter, shake Flour on it, then roll it like a Collar, double it up at both Ends, that they meet in the Middle : Roll it
out

out the fame Way, and put it up as before, till all the Butter is in it.

Pafte for any raifed Pies.

TO half a Peck of Flour, take two Pound of Butter; boil it in a Chopin of Water, make a Hole in the Flour, and pour in the Butter and Water, don't let the Sediment at the Bottom go in: Skim it clean, then work it up to a Pafte, and before it is quite cold, raife it up into any Shape you pleafe, either fmall or great Pies; if the Pafte is not wet enough, boil Water, and put in it. Do the fame in all ftanding Pafte.

Another Sort of Pafte.

TAKE half a Peck of Flour, and boil a Pound of Butter, and half a Pound of render'd Mutton Sewet in a Chopin of Water; wet it with it, and work it well while it is hot; raife it into any Shape for Pafties or Pies you pleafe; it ftands better with the Sewet mixed with Butter, than all Butter, but let it be very fweet.

A Pafte of Dripings.

TAKE a Pound and a half of Dripings, boil it in Water, and ftrain it; then let it cool, and take off the Fat, fcrape it, and boil it fo for four or five Times, then work it well up into three Pounds of Flour, and wet it with cold Water till it is a Pafte. It will be a very good Pye Cruft, or if you wet the Flour with it and boiling Water, it will make raifed Pies, but you muft raife it while it is very hot.

Cold Water Pafte for Pafties.

LAY down half a Peck of Flour, wet it with two Eggs and cold Water, work it in a Pafte, then roll it out, and put over it a Pound and a Quarter of Butter, and flour it, then roll it like a Collar, and roll it again: Do that five or fix Times, till you fee the Butter is
well

well mixed with the Pafte, then you may cover any Sort of Pies with it.

Pafte for Tarts.

TAKE a Pound of Flour, and rub it in a Quarter of a Pound of Butter, and a little fine Sugar, wet it with an Egg, and as much Water as will make it into Pafte; then roll it into what Form you pleafe for Tarts or Puddings.

To make Apple Tarts.

PARE two Oranges thin, and boil them in Water till they are tender; then fhread them fmall, and pare twenty Pipins, quarter and core them, and put to them as much Water as will cover them, then put them on the Fire, and turn them foftly, then put in half a Pound of Sugar, and the Orange-peel that was fhred, and the Juice of the Orange, and let them boil till they are pretty thick; when they are cold, put them in your Crufts, with open Pafte over them, glaze them with the White of an Egg, and grated Sugar, then bake them a light brown.

Goofe-berry Tarts.

PUT Pafte in the Patties, and give the Goofe-berries a Scald, when they are cold, put them in the Patties, with Sugar under and over them; cover them with nicked Pafte, and glaze them as before. Bake them in a flow Oven

Prune Tarts.

STEW a Pound of Prunes, with a little Sugar and Water, ftone fome of them, and put in fome of them without ftoning: Put Puff Pafte under them and over them, with a little of the Liquor they were ftewed in, fo bake them, Glaze all Tarts as in the firft Receipt of Tarts. You may ftew the Prunes in Claret, if you pleafe.

Chefnut

Chefnut Tarts.

ROAST the Chefnuts, peel them, and put Pafte in the Patties; then put in your Chefnuts, and between every *two* Chefnuts, put a Bit of Marrow rolled in Eggs, and fome Orange and Lemon-peel cut fmall; then make a Cuftard, and put it over them; bake them a little, then fend them up hot or cold.

To make Sweet-meat Tarts.

PUT Puff Pafte in the Bottom of the Patties, then put into them any Sort of preferv'd Fruit, then cut Pafte in any Shape you pleafe, or crofs bar them; then glaze them, and put them in a flow Oven for a Quarter of an Hour. When the Pafte is done, they are enough.

To keep Goofeberries for Tarts.

TAKE the Goofe-berries before they are full grown, but come to their Tafte; pick them off the Stems, then put them in Bottles that are very clean and dry, cork them very clofs, put them in a flow Oven, and when they turn white, they are enough; then rofin the Corks, and keep them in Sand: When you are going to ufe them, boil them in a Syrup, and when they are cold, put them in Puff Pafte, and cut Holes in the Top, bake them in a flow Oven. You may keep red and black Currants the fame Way.

Peach Tarts.

TAKE half ripe Peaches and pare them, and flice them in two, and take out the Stones, put fome fine powdered Sugar in the Bottom of a Stew-pan, place your Peaches in it, put them over the Fire, and ftir them often, then put Pafte in the Patty-pans, and when the Peaches are cold put them in the Patties with the Syrup they were boiled in, cover them with rich Pafte, and bake them in a flow Oven; put the Kernels of the Peaches in the Tarts. You may do Apricocks the fame Way.

Rafpberry

Raspberry Tarts.

PUT Paste in the Patties, then lay in the Raspberries, strew over them some fine Sugar; cover and bake them in a slow Oven: When they are cold, you may put Cream on them. You may make Tarts the same Way of all Sorts of Fruit, but put a carved Paste Lid on them.

To make Orange Tarts.

BOIL the Skins of two bitter Oranges in four or five Waters, till all the Bitterness is off them, and the Skin is so tender that you may thrust a Straw in them, then drain them, and pound them and six Ounces of fine Sugar into a Paste, with some of the Juice of the Oranges, and some Pipins shred small, mix it all together, and put it into your Patty-pans with Paste under them, and cross Bars over them; put them in the Oven, half an Hour bakes them. You may make Lemon Tarts the same Way.

To make Orange Cheese-cakes.

BOIL the Skins of three Oranges in five or six Waters, till the Bitterness is off them, then pound them very fine, with half a Pound of fine Sugar, beat the Yolks of eight Eggs and two Whites, till they are very thick and white; then mix the Oranges with them, and eight Ounces of oiled Butter: Put Paste in the Patty pans, and half fill them; half an Hour bakes them in a slow Oven. Lemon Cheese cakes are made the same Way, but you need not shift the Water they are boiled in, and put the Grate of an Orange or Lemon in them: Put a little Brandy in both.

To make Cheese-cakes.

TAKE two Chopins of Cream or good Milk, and the Yolks of three Eggs, and four of the Whites, beat them very well; mix them with the Milk, and set it on the Fire, when it boils take it off and drain the Whey gently from it, put to the Curd grated Nutmeg
beat

beat Cinnamon, and three Spoonfuls of Rofe water, as much Malaga, fome fine Sugar, four Ounces of Butter, a Quarter of pounded Bifcuits, and a Quarter of Currants, pick and wafh them; but before you put them in, blend all the reft very well together, then mix them in. You may bake them in any Shape or Cruft you pleafe.

To make Potatoe Cheefe-cakes.

BOIL and peel the Potatoes, and pound fix Ounces of them, then beat five Eggs, but three of the Whites, and mix the Potatoes with them, and four Ounces of Sugar, grated Lemon and Orange-peel, Nutmeg, and a Glafs of Brandy; then a little before you put them in the Patties, put in four Ounces of oil'd Butter almoft cold. Put Puff Pafte in the Patties under them.

To make Egg Cheefe-cakes.

BEAT two Eggs well, and thicken them with Flour, then beat three Eggs, and mix them with a Mutchkin of Cream and fix Ounces of Butter, put it on the Fire, and keep it ftirring one Way; when it is almoft boiling put in the two Eggs and Flour, keep it ftirring, and when it is boiled pretty thick, take it off the Fire, and feafon it with Sugar, Salt, grated Lemon-peel and Nutmeg, when they are cold, put in half a Pound of Currants wafh'd, pick'd and dried, put Pafte in your Patties, and bake them half an Hour.

To make Almond Cheefe-cakes.

TAKE half a Pound of Almonds, blanch and pound them, keeping them wetting with Brandy, or Rofe-water; beat five Eggs, but one White, mix them and your Almonds with fix Ounces of fine Sugar, the Grate of two Oranges or Lemon peel, fix Ounces of Butter oil'd, fkim and bottom it; then juft as they are going into the Oven put in the Butter, beat all well together, put Puff Pafte in the Patties, put a little Brandy in them,
then

then put them in the Oven. Half an Hour bakes them.

To make *Almond Custards.*

BOIL a Mutchkin of Cream with Cinnamon, and Orange or Lemon-peel in it; beat the Yolks of seven Eggs, and mix them with a little of the Cream before you boil it; then mix all together with a Quarter of a Pound of Almonds blanched and pounded, and a little Orange-flower Water; sweeten them to your Taste; put them on the Fire again, and keep it stirring one Way till it is almost boiling; then take it up, and put it in Cups; take out the Cinnamon and Peel: You may put the Cups in the Oven to colour them, or you may send them to Table as they are. Grate Nutmeg on them.

To make *Custards of Rice.*

BOIL a Mutchkin of Milk with two Ounces of fresh Butter in it, keep out a little of the Milk, and stir in it two Spoonfuls of the Powder of Rice, and two Eggs well beaten; then mix them with the boiled Milk; put in a Spoonful of Orange-flower or Rose-water; sweeten it to your Taste; put it on the Fire, and keep it stirring till it is pretty thick; boil the Rice in the Milk, before you put in the Eggs, and don't let it boil after the Eggs go in, but let it be scalding hot,

To make *Custards.*

BEAT six Eggs very well, leave out four of the Whites, mix them with a Mutchkin of Milk, the Grate of a Lemon and Nutmeg, sweeten it to your Taste, put it in Cups, and put them in a Stew-pan of cold Water on a slow Fire: Don't put as much Water in the Pan as will come over them; put it on a slow Fire; cover the Pan with the Lid, and when the Custards are stiff, take them out: You may brown them with a Salamander. You may do any Custards in Water the same Way.

Orange

Orange Cuftards.

TAKE the Juice of two *Seville* Oranges with a little of the Peel grated, and as much Sugar as will make it fweet; give it a Boil, and ftrain it, then boil a Mutchkin of Cream, with Nutmeg, Cinnamon and Sugar; thicken it with the Whites of five or fix Eggs beaten, then beat them all together, and put it in Cups.

Another Sort of Almond Cuftards.

BLANCH and pound a Handful of Almonds, then put to them a Mutchkin of Milk, prefs the Milk out, and fweeten it; then beat five Eggs, but two of the Whites, and mix them with the Milk, put it in Cups. You may put them in the Oven, or do them in a Pan with Water.

To put Sweet-meats of all Colours in Jelly.

LET your Jelly be very ftiff, and feafon it and clear it as you do other Jelly, put a little in the Bottom of the Turks-cap; let it ftand to cool, then lay it all over with different coloured whole Sweet-meats; then put on a little more Jelly, as much as will be half an Inch above the Sweet-meats; let it cool again, and lay on more, fo go on till the Bowl is filled, but there muft be an Inch of Jelly above all: When it is very cold, turn it out on an Afhet with the broad Part down.

To make a Trifle.

COVER your Afhet with Spunge Bifcuits, then pour over them a Mutchkin of Malaga, or white Wine, then a yellow Cream, then lay on it Heaps of coloured Sweet-meats; roaft fix or feven Apples, and rub them through a Search; put a little Sugar to them, and mix them with four Eggs, the Whites only, and wipe them up very high, and put this by Spoonfuls over the reft; but let a little of the Cream and Sweet-meats be feen. Raife it up as high as you can, fo fend it to the Table.

S

To

To make Burnt Cream.

BOIL a Mutchkin of Cream, and thicken it with the Yolks of eight Eggs and a Spoonful of Flour, boil Cinnamon and the Rind of an Orange in the Cream; take Care it is not curdled, sweeten it to your Taste; take a Quarter of a Pound of Loaf Sugar in a Stew-pan, and pour over it half a Gill of Water, let it boil till it ropes, and don't stir it till you take it off, then by Degrees strew it over your Ashet of Cream; brown it with a Salamander, or in the Oven.

To make Jelly of Hartshorn.

TAKE a Pound of Hartshorn, put it in a Tea Kettle with two Pints of Water, *Scots* Measure, and a Penny-worth of Isinglass, let it boil on a very slow Fire to a Pint, then strain it off and set it to cool, if it is too stiff, put in a little Water, and if too limber, put in another Penny-worth of Isinglass, and boil it better, it takes a great deal of boiling more than any other Stock for Jelly, season it with white Wine, Sugar, Lemons and Cinnamon to your Taste, put the Rind of a Lemon in it, beat the Whites of six Eggs, and whisk them in it: You must keep it stirring all the while it is on the Fire, have a thin Cloth tied on the Bottom of a Chair or Frame, boil it a Quarter of an Hour, and pour it up boiling hot; change the Bowl till you see it is clear. So put it in Glasses for your Use.

To make Calves Feet Jelly.

SCALD the Hair off them very clean, then sli them into, and let them ly in warm Water two Hours put them into a closs covered Sauce-pan with a Quarter of a Pound of Hartshorn, or Two-pence worth of Isinglass, put two Pints of Water to them, and let them boil very slow till they are all in Tavers, then put little of the Stock to cool, and if it is stiff, strain it off skim it very clean, and let it stand to settle; leave a the Settling at the Bottom; if it is too stiff put in little Water, if not boil it better: The best Way t

season

feafon Jelly is to your Tafte, but you may put a Mutchkin of Wine and four Lemons to three Mutch-kins of Stock, feafon it with Cinnamon, Sugar and the Rind of a Lemon, clear it as you do the Hartfhorn Jelly, with Whites of Eggs.

To make Blamong.

MAKE your Stock as you do for Jelly, but a great deal ftiffer; to a Mutchkin of Stock put a Quarter of a Pound of Almonds blanched and pounded very fine, fix bitter ones; as you are pounding wet them with a little Cream; boil Lemon peel and Cinnamon in your Stock, fweeten it to your Tafte, and when it is pretty warm, rub the Almonds in it very well thro' a Cloth; ftrain it, and if it is not white enough, put in a Gill of thick fweet Cream; put in a little Orange-flower Water, if you have it: You may put it either in Cups, or any Thing you pleafe, it will turn out if cold enough. Wet the Cups with Cream.

To make Leech Cream.

TAKE a Quarter of a Pound of Ifinglafs, pull it in Pieces, and put it to boil in a clofs covered Sauce-pan, with three Mutchkins of Water, let it boil on a very flow Fire, till it is all diffolved, and the half boiled a-way; put it to cool, and if it be ftiff, put to it half a Mutchkin of Cream, the Rind of a Lemon and Orange, a Stick of Cinnamon, and fweeten it to your Tafte You may whiten it with pounded Almonds, if you pleafe. It is a very pretty Supper Difh, when quite cold, ftick Bits of Marmalade of Oranges and Almonds cut like Straws in it. It is good for any one in a Decay.

To make whipt Sillabubs.

TAKE a Mutchkin of thick Cream, put to it half a Mutchkin of white Wine, the Juice of a Lemon, and grate the Rind in it; fweeten it to your Tafte, whifk it up well, fkim off the Top as you are whifking it, and

put

put it on a Sieve; then put Wine in the Glass, either white or red, and a little Sugar; then send it to Table with Tea Spoons about it.

To make Orange Cream.

PARE the Rind of three bitter Oranges, and steep them in two Gills of Water, till it has a strong Flavour of the Orange, then squeeze the Juice in it, beat the Yolks of six Eggs, but first boil your Liquor with half a Pound of fine Sugar, then mix in your Eggs by Degrees, for Fear of curdling. Let it have a Scald on the Fire, stirring it one Way. Put it in Cups or Glasses, cutting some of the Orange-peel like Threads, and hang them about the Rim.

To make Lemon Cream.

LEMON Cream is made the same Way, but with more Sugar, and two more Whites of Eggs. You must not whip the Whites much, or they will froth, and not thicken. When you mix your Liquor and Eggs, you must strain it before you put it on the Fire. It must not boil but be scalding hot, always stirring one Way. There must not be any Yolks of Eggs in this.

Maids Cream.

TAKE the Whites of five Eggs, and whisk them to a Froth, then put them in a Sauce-pan, with very fine Sugar, three Gills of Cream, a Spoonful of Orange-flower Water, and a little pounded Cinnamon: Put it on the Fire, and keep it stirring one Way all the Time. Don't let it boil, but it must be scalding hot; then put it in the Ashet, and brown it with a red hot Shovel.

To make a Rhenish Wine Cream.

PUT on the Fire a Mutchkin of Rhenish Wine, and a Stick of Cinnamon, and six Ounces of Loaf Sugar; while it is boiling, take six Eggs, whisk them very well, then whisk in the Wine by Degrees, then put it on the Fire,

Fire, and keep it whifking all the Time, till it is pretty thick. It muft not boil after the Eggs are in. Boil the Rind of an Orange or Lemon in the Wine; keep it whifking all the Time, and when it is fcalding hot, take it off, and put it in Cups, with as high a Froth as you can whifk on it. You may make any Sort of white Wine the fame Way.

To make Currant Cream.

BOIL a Mutchkin of Cream, and thicken it with two Eggs, when it is cold, put to it the Juice of a Chopin of Currants, and put the Currants in a Pan on the Fire, mafh them, and when they are thoroughly hot, ftrain out the Juice, and fweeten it to your Tafte; then mix it with the Cream, and put it in Cups. You may do Rafpberry or Strawberry Cream the fame Way. Don't let the Cream boil after you put in the Eggs at any Time, but it muft be fcalding hot.

Sack Cream.

TAKE a Chopin of Cream, put it on the Fire with the Rind of a Lemon, and when it boils, take it off; beat two Eggs, and mix the Cream with them by Degrees, ftirring them all the Time; then put it on the Fire again, and when it is fcalding hot, take it off, and ftir it one Way all the Time it is on the Fire, then take the China Bowl that you ferve it to Table in, and put the Juice of half a Lemon, and nine Spoonfuls of Sack in it, and fweeten both the Cream and Sack; then put in the Cream in the Bowl by Spoonfuls; fend it up when quite cold, and keep it ftirring till almoft cold.

To make yellow Lemon Cream.

GRATE off the Peel of four Lemons, fqueeze the Juice to it, and let it ftand five Hours, then ftrain it, and put to it the Whites of eight Eggs, and two Yolks well beaten and ftrained, a Pound of double refined Sugar, and a Gill of Rofe-water; ftir it well and fet it

on

on the Fire, keep it ſtirring one Way, don't let it boil; when it comes to Cream it is enough.

Yellow Cream.

BOIL a Mutchkin of Cream with a Stick of Cinnamon, and the Rind of an Orange, then beat up the Yolks of eight Eggs with Roſe-water, and when the Cream is almoſt cold mix the Eggs with it by Degrees, ſweeten it to your Taſte; put it on a ſlow Fire, and keep it ſtirring one Way, till it is ſcalding hot, don't let it boil, then pour it in a Bowl, keep it ſtirring for a while, then whip up the Whites of Eggs to a Snow, and put them in the Oven, or before the Fire to harden, pour the Cream in your Diſh, but take out the Orange-peel and Cinnamon; put red Currant Jelly, Marmalade of Oranges, and any different coloured Sweet-meats about the Diſh in Heaps, with the Whites of Eggs between every Heap. It is to be eaten cold.

Almond Cream.

BOIL a Chopin of Cream with Cinnamon, Lemon-peel and ſliced Nutmeg; then blanch and pound ſome Almonds with Roſe-water, then take the Whites of nine Eggs well beaten, and put them into your Almonds, then rub them very well through a fine Search, ſo thicken your Cream with them; keep it ſtirring on a ſlow Fire till it is ſcalding hot, ſweeten it to your Taſte; you may put it in a Diſh, or in Cups.

Ratafia Cream.

BOIL four Laurel Leaves in a Chopin of Cream, and beat up the Yolks of five Eggs in a little cold Cream, and mix it with the reſt, put it on the Fire, and keep it ſtirring one Way, don't let it boil, but be ſcalding hot: Then take out the Leaves and ſweeten it to your Taſte, then put it in Cups. It is to be eaten cold.

To

To make Steeple Cream.

BOIL a Chopin of Cream, with two Pints of Milk, set it to cool, and skim the Cream off it, then boil it again, and set it to cool; skim it, keep it boiling, and cooling and skimming till you have a Chopin of Cream that a Spoon will almost stand in it; take Care to stir it in the boiling, that no Brats come on it: Put in it, just as you are going to whisk it, half a Mutchkin of Malaga, a little fine Sugar, and the Juice of a Lemon; you must whisk it up very thick, and raise it up on the Ashet in the Shape of a Sugar Loaf: Strew it all over with coloured confected Carraways, and garnish it with different coloured Sweet-meats.

To make Strawberry or Raspberry Cream.

MASH them small, and boil them with an equal Weight of Loaf Sugar, when cold put to it a Mutchkin of Cream, or four or five Spoonfuls of either of them, and whisk them as you do Sillabubs. So fill your Glasses.

To make Coddlen or Goose-berry Cream.

CODDLE your Apples, till they are so soft that you will rub them thro' a Search with the Back of a Spoon, sweeten them to your Taste; when they are cold mix them with Cream: Goose-berries are done the same Way. Put them on an Ashet.

To make a very pretty red Cream.

TAKE a Mutchkin of Cream, and colour it with Cochineal: Put the Grate of an Orange and Lemon in it, a little Malaga, and the White of an Egg; sweeten it to your Taste, whip it up thick and put it in Glasses. Any one may eat it, for Cochineal is very wholsome.

To make Cream Deloutee.

TAKE a Mutchkin of Cream, the Rind of a Lemon or Orange-peel, and a Stick of Cinnamon, sweeten

ten it to your Taſte; let it ſtand till it is almoſt as cold
as new Milk, then take the yellow Skins that are in the
Gizzards of two Fowls, waſh them clean, cut them
ſmall, and put them in the Cream; then ſtrain the
Cream thro' a thin Cloth into the Aſhet, rubbing the
Cloth; ſtrain it two or three Times, ſtill keeping it rub
bing: You muſt be very quick in ſtraining it, or it will
jelly in the Cloth; then put it on warm Water, and co
ver the Aſhet, then put Fire on the Cover; when it
is jelly'd, take it off gently and ſet it to cool, then
ſerve it up: It muſt be the Skins of the Gizzards of
Hens, Chickens or Turkies.

To make Rice Cream.

TAKE three Spoonfuls of the Flour of Rice, three
Yolks of Eggs, three Spoonfuls of Water, and two
Spoonfuls of Orange-flower Water; mix them well
together, and put to them a Mutchkin of Cream, and
ſet it on the Fire; keep it ſtirring till of a right Thickneſs, then diſh it and eat it cold.

Clouted Cream.

TAKE an *Engliſh* Gallon of good new Milk, ſcald
it on a clear Fire, and keep it ſtirring; when it is at the
Boil, take it off and ſtir it a little, then put it in a
Milk pan, let it ſtand twenty four Hours, then divide
the Cream with a Knife as it ſtands upon the Pan,
and take it off with a Skimmer that the Milk may run
from it; then lay it on a Diſh, one Piece upon another,
with fine Sugar between each Piece till the Diſh is full,
keep it thus twenty four Hours before you ſpread it
If you pleaſe beat Part of it with a little Roſe-water,
and a Lair of it, and a Lair of unbeaten Clouts, with
Sugar between, this clouted Cream beaten with a
Spoon till it is thick and light, makes *Spaniſh* Cream.
It muſt be done with a little Roſe-water and Sugar.

Sack

Sack Cream.

BOIL a Bottle of white Wine, a little Cinnamon and Sugar to your Taste; then beat four Eggs with a little Nutmeg, and mix in the Wine by Degrees, keeping the Eggs beating all the Time; then put it on the Fire and keep it whisking, don't let it boil, but scalding hot; put it in Caudle Cups, send it hot to Table with a great Froth whisked on it, if you like it stiff and cold, put in the Yolks of eight Eggs, and two Whites.

To make Tablets.

WET a Pound of double refined Sugar, with two Gills of Water, it must be very finely pounded; put it on the Fire, and keep it stirring all the Time till the Drop stands on the Spoon; and when it begins to candy about the Sides of the Pan, it is enough. Oil a Dish, and just as you are going to pour it out, put in it two Tea Spoonfuls of the Oil of Cinnamon, keeping it always stirring till you pour it on the Dish: When almost cold, cut it in any Shape you please. Ginger Tablets are made the same Way; but instead of the Oil of Cinnamon, put in two Drops of Ginger, beaten and sifted very fine.

To make a Crokain.

TAKE three Quarters of a Pound of fine Sugar, put it in a clear Copper-pan with two Gills of Water; put it on the Fire, let it boil slow, skim it, but don't stir it, put in the Juice of half a Lemon, then let it boil brown, then take a Spoon and try if it ropes; oil your Mold, and spin it on as neatly as you can, and let it be pretty thick at the Bottom, when it is done, take it off as gently as you can. You may put any of the Creams mentioned in this Book, or red or green preserved Apples or Oranges under it.

T

To make a floating Island.

TAKE half a Pound of Currant Jelly, and the Whites of four Eggs; put them in a large Bowl, and whisk it till it is as thick that you may drop it with a Spoon into any Shape you please: You must keep whisking all one Way, it takes a long Time to whisk it, and it must be whisked from the Bottom of the Bowl; then drop it by Spoonfuls in an Asher, and raise it up as high as you can; put under it two Gills of Cream, a Spoonful of Rose-water, and a little Sugar: You may make it of roasted Apples the same Way, but they must be cold, and mash them with the Back of a Spoon. You may put a yellow Cream under it, but don't make it too stiff.

Solid Sillabubs.

TAKE a Chopin of very thick Cream, put into it three Gills of Malaga, the Grate of a Lemon, the Juice of two bitter Oranges, and sweeten it to your Taste, beat it well together for a Quarter of an Hour, then skim it with a Spoon, and put it in Glasses.

To make Sillabubs from the Cow.

SWEETEN either Wine, Cedar, or strong Ale, put it in a Bowl, take it to the Cow, and milk her on your Liquor as fast as you can. You may make it at home, by warming it, and pour it on the Liquor out of a Tea Pot.

A Jelly Posset.

TAKE twelve Eggs, leave out half the Whites, and beat them very well, put them into a large Bowl or a Soup Dish, with a Mutchkin of Malaga or strong Ale, sweeten it to your Taste, and set it on a Pan or Pot of boiling Water, keeping it stirring all the Time, then have ready a Chopin of Milk or Cream, boiled with Cinnamon and Nutmeg, and when your Wine and Eggs are scalding hot, put the Milk to them boiling hot, then

take

take it off the Fire, and cover it for half an Hour, so
send it up.

A Sack Posset, or what is called the Snow Posset.

BOIL a Chopin of Cream or Milk with Cinnamon
and Nutmeg; then beat the Yolks of ten Eggs, and
mix them with a little cold Milk; then by Degrees mix
them with the Cream, stir it on the Fire till it is scalding hot; sweeten it to your Taste, put in your Dish a
Mutchkin of Sack, with some Sugar and Nutmeg, set
it on a Pot of boiling Water, and when the Wine is hot,
let one take the Cream, and another the Whites of
Eggs: The Whites must be beaten with a little Sack.

To make Oat-meal Flummery.

PUT three large Handfuls of Oat-meal ground
small in two Chopins of Water: Let it steep a Day and
a Night, then pour off the clear Water, and put two
Chopins more on it, and let it stand the same Time,
then stir it, and strain it through a Hair Sieve, till it is
as Porridge, that is, what is called in *England* Hasty Pudding, stir it all the Time, that it may be extremely
smooth before you set it on the Fire, put in a Spoonful of Sugar, and two of Orange-flower Water, when it
is boiled enough, pour it in a shallow Dish, when cold,
you may eat it with Wine and Sugar, Ale or Milk.

To make Scots Flummery.

TAKE a Mutchkin of Milk, and one of Cream;
beat the Yolks of nine Eggs, with a little Rose-water,
Sugar and Nutmeg; put it in a Dish, and the Dish o-
ver a Pan of boiling Water covered close, when it begins to grow thick, have ready some Currants plumped in Sack, and strew over it. It must not be stirred
while it is over the Fire, and when it is pretty stiff,
send it up hot.

To make *Weft Country Flummery.*

LAY half a Peck of Wheat Brawn in Steep, in cold Water, for three or four Days; then ftrain it, and boil it to a Jelly, fweeten it with Sugar, and put in either Orange-fiower, or Rofe-water; then fet it to cool, and eat it with Cream, Milk, Wine or Beer.

To make a *Hedge-hog.*

BLANCH and beat a Pound of Almonds very fine, with a Spoonful of Sack or Orange-flower Water, to keep them from oiling; make it into a ftiff Pafte, then beat fix Eggs, and put two Whites, fweeten it with fine Sugar, then put in half a Mutchkin of Cream, and a Quarter of a Pound of beat Butter, fet it on your Stove, and keep it ftirring till it is ftiff, that you make into the Shape of a Hedge hog, then ftick it full of blanched Almonds cut in Straws, fet them on it like the Briftles, with two Currants plump'd for Eyes, then place it in the Middle of the Difh, and boil fome Cream; put in it the Yolks of two Eggs, and fweeten it to your Tafte, put it on a flow Fire, and when it is fcalding hot take it off, you muft keep it ftirring all the while; when it is cold put it about the Hedge-hog.

To make *Flummery Caudle.*

TAKE a Mutchkin of fine Oat-meal, put to it two Chopins of Water, let it ftand twelve Hours, then ftrain it into a Skellet with a little Mace and Nutmeg, fet it on the Fire and keep it ftirring, and let it boil a Quarter of an Hour, if it is too thick put in more Water, and let it boil longer, add to it a Mutchkin of white Wine, the Juice of a Lemon or Orange, and a Bit of Butter. Sweeten it to your Tafte, let it have one Boil. You may put in the Yolks of two Eggs, but let it boil after you put in the Eggs, let it be fcalding hot, keep it ftirring till you difh it.

To make Hartshorn Flummery.

TAKE a Mutchkin of very stiff Hartshorn Jelly, and put to it two Gills of Cream, Nutmeg, Cinnamon, Lemon-peel and two Laurel Leaves, sweeten it to your Taste, boil all together in a clean Sauce-pan; then strain it in large Cups, and when cold, turn it out in a Dish; put Cream, Sugar and Wine about them.

To make a Calf's Foot Flummery.

TAKE four Calf's Feet, split them, and take out the long Bone, put them in three Chopins of Water, with some Cinnamon, Mace, Nutmeg and Lemon-peel, let it boil gently till it is a strong Jelly; set it to cool, and skim off all the Fat, but strain it first; when cold take the Sediment, put it in the Pan with a Mutchkin of Cream, sweeten it to your Taste, put it over the Fire; take the Yolks of eight Eggs and beat them very well with a little cold Cream, when the Jelly is lukewarm, put in the Eggs, keep it stirring till the Eggs begin to be set, sweeten it to your Taste; then run it thro' a Sieve, and put it in Cups. It is to be eaten cold.

A Sack or Ale Posset.

BOIL a Chopin of Cream or new Milk, and grate in five or six fine Biscuits, and let them boil with the Cream, season it with Sugar and Nutmeg, let it stand a little to cool, then put half a Mutchkin of Sack or strong Ale in your Dish or Bowl: Let it be a little hot, then hold up your Hand pretty high, and pour in the Cream: Let it stand a little, then send it up.

A Sack Posset without Cream or Eggs.

TAKE a Pound of *Jordan* Almonds, lay them all Night in Water, then blanch and beat them very fine, with a Gill of Orange-flower Water, and put them in a Chopin of Water with the Crumbs of a Penny Loaf, beat Cinnamon, Nutmeg and Sugar; let it boil till it be pretty thick, keep it stirring all the Time, then warm

two

two Gills of Sack and put to it, ſtir all together; ſerve it up hot.

A very good Poſſet.

TAKE a Chopin of Cream, and mix it with a Mutchkin of ſtrong Ale, then beat the Yolks of eight Eggs, and three of the Whites, then put them to the Cream and Ale; ſweeten it to your Taſte, and grate Nutmeg in it; ſet it over the Fire, and keep it ſtirring all the while, when it is thick, and before it boils, take it off and put it in the Diſh very gently, ſo ſend it up, ſtir all Things but one Way that have Eggs in them.

To make an Oat-meal Poſſet.

TAKE a Mutchkin of Milk, boil it with Nutmeg and Cinnamon, and put in it two Spoonfuls of Flour of Oat-meal, and boil it till the Rawneſs is off the Oat-meal; then take three Spoonfuls of Sack, and three of Ale, and two of Sugar; ſet it over the Fire till it is ſcalding hot, then put them to the Milk, give it one Stir, and let it ſtand on the Fire a Minute or two, and pour it in your Bowl; cover it and let it ſtand a little, then ſend it up.

Egg Cheeſe.

TAKE a Chopin of Milk, a Mutchkin of Cream beat, and ten Eggs; leave out four Whites, mix them well with the Cream, Lemon-peel, Cinnamon, Sugar, Roſe-water, and half a Mutchkin of white Wine, then ſet it on the Fire, and keep it ſtirring all the Time till it boils; when you ſee it broke, take it off and put it in any ſhaped Mold that has Holes in it, till the Whey runs out; when cold put it on the Diſh: You may put Wine and Sugar on them, or you may boil two Gills of Cream, thicken it with the Yolks of two Eggs, and pour it about it.

Cheeſe Loaves.

TAKE three Chopins of Milk, put a Spoonful of Runnet in it, and when it is come, preſs the Whey gently out of it; then put as much grated Bread as Curd, and the Yolks of twelve Eggs, fix Whites, two Gills of Cream, beat Cinnamon, Mace, Nutmeg, Sugar, two Spoonfuls of Flour, a little Salt and a Glass of Sack or Brandy; make it into a Paste, roll fome of it thin to fry, make the reft in a Loaf, and bake it, then cut a Hole in the Top, pour in fome beat Butter, Cream and Sugar; put the fried Cakes about it in the Difh, and fend it up hot.

Almond Puffs.

BLANCH two Ounces of Almonds, then take their Weight of fine Loaf Sugar, beat them together with Orange-flower Water, then whip up the Whites of three Eggs and put to them, and add as much fifted Sugar as will make it into a Paste; then make it into little Cakes, and bake them in a very flow Oven.

Pudding Puffs.

TAKE half a Mutchkin of Cream and three well beaten Eggs, three Spoonfuls of Flour, two Spoonfuls of Rofe-water, Sugar, Nutmeg and a little Salt; mix all well together; butter fome Cups, and fill them more than half full of it, and bake them ten Minutes in a flow Oven: When they are done, turn them out on a Difh, and grate Sugar on them; fend them up hot.

Lemon Puffs.

BEAT and fift a Pound of Loaf Sugar, mix it with the Juice of two Lemons, and the Rind grated fine, whifk the Whites of three Eggs to a Snow; then beat all together very well, fift Sugar on Papers, and drop it on by Spoonfuls, don't let them be too near one another, put them in a very flow Oven. You may make Orange Puffs the fame Way.

Orange Loaves.

CUT a Bit out of the End of the Oranges, and take out all the Infide, and grate them; boil them in
different

different Waters till they are tender, and all the Bitternefs off them; let them dry, and boil them in a thin
Syrup, till it has penetrated through them very well,
then let them ftand in the Syrup a Day or two, then
take the Yolks of fix Eggs, two Whites, a Quarter of
a Pound of fine Bifcuits pounded, Butter, two Gills
of Cream, fome of the Grate of the Orange, Sugar,
and Nutmeg, put it in a Pan, and ftir it on the Fire
till it is thick, then ftir in it a little Brandy, and fill the
Orange Skins, bake and ferve them up, with beat
Butter, Wine and Sugar in a Cup.

To make Wafers.

LET the Flour be very dry; make it in a thick
Batter with Cream; feafon it with Sugar and Cinnamon, and a very little Salt; beat an Egg very well,
and put in it; butter your Irons, and let them be very
hot, then put in a Tea Spoonful of the Batter, clap
the Irons together, and hold them on the Fire for half
a Minute, turning them; then take out the Wafer, and
give it a Turn round your Finger, till it is in the Shape
of a Funnel, as faft as you make them lay them on
a Difh before the Fire.

Dutch *Wafers.*

BEAT four Eggs very well, mix with them a
Pound of Flour, a Mutchkin of Cream, twelve Ounces of beat Butter, feafon it with Sugar, Nutmeg and
Rofe water, put in two Spoonfuls of Barm, mix all
well together, and bake them in your Wafer-irons;
there muft be more of the Batter put in thefe than
the other Wafers, and they take a longer Time on the
Fire.

To make a Hen's Neft.

TAKE Calves Feet Jelly that is very ftrong, and put
it in a white Bowl or a Turks-cap, fill it near half full
of the Jelly, let it be cold, take five Eggs, make a Hole

in the narrow End of them, that the Yolks and Whites may come out; then fill them with Blamong: Let them ſtand till they are cold, then take off the Shells by Pieces, and take care not to break the Blamong; then lay them in the Middle of the Jelly, ſo that they don't touch one another; then pour more Jelly on them when it is almoſt cold: Cut ſome Lemon-peel as Straws, and when the Jelly is ſtiff, ſtrew it over it; then pour a little more Jelly over it: When all is cold and very ſtiff, dip the Bowl in hot Water; have an Aſhet ready, and put it on the Top of the Bowl, and turn it out quick: Don't let the Bowl be a Moment in the Water.

To make a Caudle for ſweet Pies.

TAKE two Gills of white Wine, a little Nutmeg, Sugar, and Lemon-peel, put it on the Fire, and when it is ſcalding hot, beat the Yolks of two Eggs, and mix them with a little cold Wine, then mix all together; keep it ſtirring till it is ſcalding hot, then take it up, and pour it over the Pye or Tart.

To make Fairy Butter.

TAKE the Yolks of four hard Eggs, and half a Pound of Loaf ſugar beat and ſifted, half a Pound of freſh Butter, bray them in a clean Bowl with two Spoonfuls of Orange-flower Water; when it is well mixed, force it through the Corner of a thin Canvas Strainer in little Heaps on a Plate. It is a very pretty Supper Diſh.

To make a Slipcoat Cheeſe.

TAKE two *Engliſh* Gallons of hot Milk, juſt milked, and put to it twelve Spoonfuls of Runnet, and when it comes, put a thin Cloth in a Cheeſe-vat; then take out the Curd with a Saucer, and lay them as gently as you can; then pour a little Water ſoftly on the Curd, and let all the Whey run out; then put on more Curd and more Water; do this till the Vat is

U   quite

quite full, then put a Cloth over it, and a thin Board,
and when it falls put more Curd to it, and lay a Pound
Weight on the Board: This Quantity makes two Cheeses ; let it lye in the Vat ten Hours, then turn it with
a dry Cloth, and put it in the Vat again, and let it ly
ten Hours more ; then turn it on a dry Board, and
sprinkle a little Salt on it ; let it ly till the Salt is melted, then get Nettles, pluck off the Leaves and wipe
them clean ; spread them on a dry Board, and lay the
Cheese on them, then cover it with them, and let it
be kept in a warm Place : Change the Nettle Leaves
twice a Day, wiping the Cheese every Time with a
soft Cloth. It will be ripe in ten Days, or a Fortnight.

To make Cream Cheese, as at Newport.

GET a Vat, a Quarter and a half high, the Bottom
and Top must not be fastened, it must be four Square,
with Holes all over, then take two Chopins of Cream,
six Chopins of new Milk, and set it with Runnet,
when it is come, put a dry Cloth in the Vat, and lay
' the Curd in it with a China Saucer, and put it into the
Vat, strew a little Salt in two or three Lairs till all the
Curd is in, cover it and press it as other Cheeses,
let it stand two or three Days till all the Whey is out,
but turn it with dry Cloths every Day, then salt it
lightly two Days, let it dry without rubbing. It is
to be made in *May*.

To make a good Cheese.

TAKE three Chopins of Milk hot from the Cow, and
a Chopin of Cream, put one Spoonful of Runnet in
it, and when it comes, break it and put in a little
Salt, put a Cloth in the Vat, then put in the Curd,
and press it as you do other Cheese ; turn it in the
Vat often, and when it is wheyed, salt it, then put it
to dry, wiping and turning it every Day. You must
not cut it till it is a Year old.

To

To make a thick Cheese.

TAKE the Milk of ten Cows, and put to it three Spoonfuls of Runnet, and when it comes, break it and whey it, and let it ly for a while; then whey it again, and when it is very well wheyed, break into it two Pounds of sweet Butter, and a little Salt; then put it in the Vat, and press it very well; turn it very often, and change the Cloths: You may put wet Cloths at first about it, and thereafter put dry Cloths; let it ly fourteen Hours in the Press, then take it out and salt it a little, then dry it with a Cloth. Put it on a dry Board, and wipe and turn it every Day.

To make a Welsh Rabbet.

CUT Toasts, and toast them on both Sides, then toast the Cheese on the Bread, and send it up hot.

To toast Cheese.

TOAST the Bread and sock it in Wine, set it before the Fire, cut the Cheese in very thin Slices, rub Butter over the Bottom of a Plate, lay the Cheese in, pour in two or three Spoonfuls of Wine, cover it with another Plate, set it on a Chaffing-dish of Coals for three Minutes, then mix it, and when it is done, lay it on the Bread, brown it with a Salamander, or a red hot Shovel.

To toast Cheese another Way.

TAKE a Quarter of a Pound of *Cheshire* Cheese, not too fat, two Ounces of Butter, and two Eggs; beat all together very well, then prepare some Toasts pretty brown, butter them on both Sides, then spread the Cheese upon them: Then brown it with a Salamander, or a red hot Fire shovel. Serve it up hot.

To make Wigs.

TAKE a Quarter of a Peck of Flour, rub into it three Quarters of a Pound of Butter, something more than

than Half a Pound of Sugar, a little Nutmeg and Ginger grated, three Eggs well beaten; put to them half a Mutchkin of thick Barm, and a Glass of Brandy, make a Hole in your Flour, and pour all in, with as much warm Milk as will make it in a light Paste; let it stand before the Fire to rise Half an Hour, then make it into a Dozen and a Half of Wigs.   Bake them Half an Hour.

A Plumb-cake or Bun.

TAKE five Pounds of Flour, and put to it half an Ounce of Nutmegs, Cloves and Mace, finely beaten, and a little Salt, mix all well together, then take a Chopin of Milk, let it boil, put into it three Pounds of Butter; when melted, and blood warm, mix it with a Chopin of Barm, and two Gills of Brandy, twenty Eggs well beaten, ten Whites, six Pounds of well clean'd Currants; mix in the Flour, make a Hole in the Middle of your Flour, and put in the Milk and other Things, mixing it well with your Hands, cover it warm before the Fire to rise, then put it in the Hoop, if the Oven is hot, two Hours will bake it; you may put Sweet-meats in it if you please.

To make Wigs another Way.

TAKE two Pounds of Flour, and a Quarter of a Pound of Butter, and as much Sugar, Nutmeg, Cloves and Mace, of each a little, pound in them a Quarter of an Ounce of Carraway Seeds, a little Barm in as much Cream as will make it in Paste, mix all together, and work them well; set them by the Fire to rise; when the Oven is ready they will soon bake.

To make Bath Buns.

TAKE two Pounds of Flour, a Mutchkin of Barm, put a little Brandy in the Barm, and three Eggs well beaten, a little warm Milk, Nutmeg and a little Salt, rub into the Flour a Pound of Butter, and a Pound of confected Carraways, mix all together, and work it with
                                                        your

your Hands; fet them before the Fire to rife; bake
them in a quick Oven, on flour'd Papers, in what
Shape you pleafe.

To make Shrewsbury Cakes.

TAKE one Pound of Sugar, three Pounds of Flour,
a Nutmeg and fome Cinnamon beaten, the Sugar and
Spice muft be fifted in the Flour; wet it with three
Eggs, and as much melted Butter as will make it in a
good Thicknefs, to roll into a Pafte; mould it well,
aud roll it and cut it into what Shape you pleafe:
Prick them before they go into the Oven.

To make Almond Cakes.

TAKE a Pound of Almonds, blanch and beat them
very well, with a little Orange-flower Water, beat
three Eggs, but two Whites, and put to them a Pound
of Sugar fifted; and then put in your Almonds, and
beat all together very well: Butter white Paper, and
lay your Cakes in what Form you pleafe, and bake
them.

To make Drop Bifcuit.

TAKE eight Eggs and a Pound of fine Sugar
pounded and fifted, and twelve Ounces of fine Flour
well dried; beat your Eggs well, then put in your
Sugar, and beat it, and then your Flour by Degrees,
and beat it all together for an Hour without ceafing.
Your Oven muft be as hot as for Penny Bread. Then
flour fome Paper, and drop your Bifcuits into what Bignefs you pleafe, and put them into the Oven as faft
as you can, and when you fee them rife, watch them,
and if they begin to colour, take them out again, and
put in more, and if the firft is not enough put them in
again: If they are right done they will have a white
Ice on them, you may put in Carraway-feeds if you
pleafe. When they are all baked, put them into the
Oven again, till they are very dry.

To make Marlborough *Cakes.*

TAKE eight Eggs, beat them, and put to them a Pound of Sugar beaten and fifted, beat it three Quarters of an Hour together; then put in three Quarters of a Pound of fine dry Flour, and two Ounces of Carraway-feeds, beat it all well together, and bake it in a quick Oven in Tin Pans.

A Seed-cake.

TAKE two Pounds of fine Flour well dried, and rub in it a Pound of frefh Butter and ten Eggs, leaving out five Whites, three Spoonfuls of Cream, four Spoonfuls of good Barm; mix all well together, and fet it to the Fire, but not too near, when it is well rifen, put in a Pound of confected Carraway. An Hour and a Quarter will bake it.

Another Sort of little Cakes.

TAKE a Pound of Flour, a Pound of Butter, and rub the Butter in the Flour, two Spoonfuls of Barm, and two Eggs: Make it up in a Pafte buttered Paper: Roll your Pafte out the Thicknefs of a Crown: Cut them out with the Top of a Tin Canifter: Sift fine Sugar over them, and bake them in a flow Oven for an Hour.

To make Whetftone *Cakes.*

TAKE half a Pound of fine Flour, and half a Pound of Loaf Sugar, pounded and fearched, a Spoonful of Carraway Seeds, the Yolk of an Egg, and the Whites of three; a little Rofe or Orange-flower Water: Mix all together, and roll it out as thin as a Wafer; cut them with a Glafs, lay them on floured Papers, and bake them in a flow Oven.

A Seed-cake very rich.

TAKE a Pound of Flour dried, a Pound of Sugar beaten and fifted, a Pound of Butter work'd with your Hand to a Cream: Beat the Yolks of ten Eggs, fix

Whites,

Whites, and mix all together; an Ounce of Carraway Seeds, and a Gill of Brandy. Keep it beating till you put it in the Oven.

To make a Plumb-cake.

TAKE four Pounds of fine Flour well dried, five Pounds of Currants well picked and rubbed, five Pounds of Butter beat to a Cream, two Pounds of Almonds beaten fine, thirty four Eggs, half the Whites, two Pounds of fine Sugar beaten and sifted, beaten Mace, Cloves, Ginger, Nutmeg and two Gills of Brandy: Beat your Sugar first in your Butter, then all the rest by Degrees. You may put in Orange, Lemon-peel candied, and Citron. Keep it beating till you put it in the Oven: Four Hours will bake it.

To ice a great Cake.

TAKE two Pounds of the finest double refined Sugar, and beat and sift it, beat and sift a little Stearch, and mix with it; beat six Whites of Eggs to a Froth, and put to it some Gum-water, then mix and beat all this together two Hours, and put it on your Cake, when it is baked, set it in the Oven a Quarter of an Hour.

A rich Nun's Cake.

TAKE four Pounds of fine Flour, and three Pounds of fine Sugar pounded and sifted, dry both by the Fire, beat four Pounds of Butter with your Hands to a Cream; then beat thirty five Eggs, leaving out half the Whites, and beat them and the Butter together, till all appears like Butter. Put in a Gill of Brandy, and beat it again; then take your Flour and Sugar, with six Ounces of Carraway Seeds, and strew it in by Degrees, beating it all the Time for two Hours together. Butter your Hoop, and let it stand three Hours in a moderate Oven.

Sugar Bifcuits.

TAKE fix Dozen of Eggs, and break them all, keep out one Dozen and a half of the Whites, then take and beat them till they drop like Water; then put in by Degrees half a Stone of Sugar well beat and fearched; then beat it till it be extraordinary white and thick. You may know when it is enough, for there will be no red Strings through it; then put in it two Gills of Brandy, and a Quarter of a Pound of Carraway Seeds, then ftir in fix Fourths of Flour, then drop it upon your Papers, then glaze the Bifcuits with fine Sugar before you put them in the Oven. See that the Oven be not too hot.

A Diet Loaf.

TAKE fix Eggs, beat them till they drop like Water, and put in twelve Ounces of fine Sugar, well beat and fearched; then put in a Spoonful or two of Brandy, and the Grate of two Lemons, mix all together, and beat it with your Whifk well, then put in ten Ounces of Flour, then rub the Frame with Butter. let it ftand an Hour in the Oven. Paper the Top, that it may not burn.

To make Saffron Cakes.

TAKE three Pounds of the fineft Flour, and dry it before the Fire, mix in it when it is cold, three Quarters of a Pound of fine powdered Sugar, make a Hole in the Middle of the Flour, beat fix Eggs very well and pour them in the Hole, take a Quarter of an Ounce of Saffron, dry and powder it, put it in a Mutchkin of Milk, with half a Pound of Butter, warm it on the Fire, and when the Butter is melted take it off, let it be but juft warm: When you pour it to the Flour, whifk among the Eggs three Gills of very good Barm, then put in the Milk and beat it together with your Handss, fhake a little Flour on it, and cover it by the Fire till it rifes, then mould it in Cakes the Bignefs of Bakes: They muft have as flow an Oven as

Milk

Milk-bakes, and if they are too ſtiff, you muſt put in a little more Milk.

To make Ratafia Biſcuits.

POUND and ſift a Pound and three Quarters of Loaf Sugar, blanch and beat to a Paſte a Pound of bitter Almonds, mix half the Sugar with them, as you are pounding the Almonds keep them wet with Roſe-water, beat the Whites of ſix Eggs to Snow, and mix the reſt of the Sugar with them: Then juſt as you are going to put them in the Oven mix all together; drop them on flour'd Papers, a Spoonful in a Place. The Oven muſt not be very hot.

To make ſhort Bread.

TAKE a Peck of Flour, make a Hole in the Middle, melt three Pounds of good Butter in a Mutchkin of Barm, put Carraway or what dry Sweet-meats you pleaſe in the Flour; then pour in your Butter and Barm, work it well with your Hands, and if too dry, put in a little warm Water; when it is well worked, roll it out in Cakes of what Shape you pleaſe, prick it well with a Fork, and bake it on floured Papers.

To make a Seed Cake.

BEAT ſixteen Ounces of good Butter to a Cream, with your Hands, pound and ſift ſixteen Ounces of Sugar, beat twelve Eggs, the Yolks and Whites ſeparate, a Pound of fine Flour well dried, put in all theſe by Spoonfuls, keeping the Butter beating all the Time, the Yolks muſt be beat to Cream, the Whites to a Snow. Don't put in the thin that will fall to the Bottom of the Whites of the Eggs; beat in half an Ounce of Carraway Seeds; when it is beat enough it will come eaſy off your Hands, put it in your Hoop, two Hours bakes it in not too ſlow an Oven.

To

To make Biscuits.

TAKE fifteen Eggs, beat them till they drop like water off the Whisk, then beat two Pounds of Sugar, and sift it; put in your Sugar by Degrees, and the Grate of an Orange or Lemon, or Carraway Seed, a Pound and an half of Flour, stir all together, drop them by Spoonfuls on floured Paper; don't let the Oven be too hot.

To make white Cakes.

TAKE three Chopins of fine Flour, a Pound and a half of Butter, and a Mutchkin of Cream, two Gills of good Barm, a Gill of Rose water and Brandy, a little Mace and Nutmegs beaten, nine Eggs, four Whites well beaten, five Ounces of fine Sugar, mix the Sugar and Spice, and a very little Salt with your dry Flour, and keep out a Handful of the Flour, melt the Butter in a little Cream: When a little cold, put the Eggs and Barm in it, make a Hole in the Midst, and pour in all the Flour, stirring it round with your Hand all one Way till well mixed; strew on the Flour you left out, and set it before the Fire to rise, cover'd with a Cloth: Have three Pounds of Currants well wash'd, pick'd and dried; mingle them in the Flour before you wet it; butter your Hoop, set it in a quick Oven, or it will not rise. An Hour and a half bakes it.

To make the thin Dutch Biscuits.

TAKE five Pounds of Flour, and two Ounces of Carraway Seed, half a Pound of Sugar, and some more than a Mutchkin of Milk, put into it three Qurters of a Pound of Butter, warm the Milk, and put in a Mutchkin of good Barm, make a Hole in the Middle of your Flour, and pour all in, and make it in a Paste, and let it stand a Quarter of an Hour by the Fire to rise; then mold it and roll it in Cakes pretty thin; prick them all over pretty much, or they will blister. Bake them a Quarter of an Hour.

To

To make Quince Cakes.

TAKE two Pounds of dried Flour, beat sixteen Ounces of sweet Butter with your Hands till it is in a Cream; then beat twelve Eggs, but half the Whites; pound and sift fourteen Ounces of fine Sugar, wash, dry and pick twelve Ounces of Currants, then mix them all by Degrees, keeping them beating all the Time; put in Nutmeg, Cinnamon and Brandy; when they are beat enough, the Dough will come clean off your Hands; then butter some Tart Pans, and bake them not in too hot an Oven, but keep the Oven-door clofs while they are baking. You may make small Seed-cakes the same Way.

York *Cakes.*

TAKE half a Peck of Flour, a Mutchkin of Barm, two Pound of Currants, a Pound of Butter, rub it into the Flour, grate two Nutmegs in it; mix all together with a little Salt and some Sugar, wet it with hot Water, it will make twelve Cakes, but let it ly before the Fire to rise. Bake them in a quick Oven.

To make Naples *Biscuits.*

TAKE a Pound of fine Sugar pounded and sifted, a Pound of fine Flour, beat eight Eggs, with two Spoonfuls of Rose-water, mix the Flour and Sugar, then wet it with the Eggs, and as much cold Water as will make a light Paste, beat the Paste very well, then put them in Tin Pans. Bake them in a gentle Oven.

To make Macaroons.

BLANCH and beat a Pound of Almonds very fine, keeping them wetting with Orange-flower Water: Take an equal Quantity of fine Sugar pounded and sifted, then beat up the Whites of eight Eggs, and mix them all together; place them handsomely on Wafers, then on Tin Plates or Papers. Bake them in a flow Oven.

To make Ginger-bread.

TAKE half a Peck of Flour well dried, five Pounds of Treacle, half a Pound of Butter, two Ounces of beaten Ginger, an Ounce of Carraway Seed; boil the Treacle and Butter together, then mix it with the Flour and Seeds: You may put candied Orange or Lemon-peel in it. If you please put three Eggs in it, bake them in little Cakes on butter'd Papers.

To make Dutch *Ginger-bread.*

MIX four Pounds of Flour, two Ounces of beaten Ginger; rub in the Flour half a Pound of Butter, and add to it two Ounces of Carraway Seeds, two of Orange peel dried and rubbed to Powder, two Pounds and a Quarter of Treacle; mix all together, and beat it with a Rolling-pin, and make it up in thirty Cakes, prick them with a Fork, and put them on double buttered Papers.

Poor Knights of Windsor.

TAKE a Roll, and cut it into Slices, soke them in Sack, then dip them in Yolks of Eggs, and fry them; serve them up with beat Butter, Sack and Sugar.

To make Buns.

TAKE two Pounds of Flour, a Mutchkin of Barm, put a little Sack in the Barm, and three Eggs well beat, knead all these together with a little warm Milk, Nutmeg and Salt, then lay it before the Fire till it rises very light, then knead in it sixteen Ounces of sweet Butter, and a Pound of confected Carraway, and bake them in a quick Oven on floured Papers, in what Shape you please.

A Cake to eat hot.

TAKE two Pounds of Flour, rub in it half a Pound of Butter, six Ounces of Sugar, grated Nutmeg and Salt, beat up four Eggs with two Gills of Barm, put as much warm Milk as will make it in a light Dough, work it well and put it to the Fire to rise: An Hour and

and a half bakes it. You may put half a Pound of Currants, and half a Pound of ston'd Raisins in it, if you please.

A common Breakfast Cake.

TAKE three Quarters of a Pound of Flour, eight Ounces of Butter, four Eggs, half an Ounce of Carraway Seeds; beat it well with your Hands, and bake it in a quick Oven.

Bath *Cakes.*

TAKE a Quart of Flour, a Pound of Butter, ten Ounces of confected Carraways, six Eggs, and but three Whites, six Spoonfuls of Barm, and a little Cream; mix all together, then put them in the Flour, the Butter and Cream must be melted, don't let it be too hot, then put it to the Barm and Eggs; work the Dough well, and set it to the Fire to rise; then shake in the Carraways, and make it into little Cakes, and bake them on floured Papers in a quick Oven.

C H A P. V.

Of PICKLING, &c.

RULES to be observed.

ALWAYS use Stone Jars for all Sorts of Pickles that require hot Pickle; for Vinegar and Salt will penetrate through all earthen Vessels: Stone and Glass are the only Things to keep Pickles in: Don't put your Hands in them, but take them up with a Spoon: Let your Brass Pan for any Pickles be very bright and clean, and your Pan for white Pickles well tinned: Use the very best Vinegar, and when they are in the Jars, and cold, melt Sewet, and when it is as cold that it will but just pour on them, put it over them, then cover them with wet Bladders.

To pickle Samphire.

IF it is fresh pulled, put it in a Pickle of Salt and Water, that will bear an Egg, changing the Water every four Days, till the Samphire is yellow; then drain it well, and put it in a Brass Kettle, with green Cabbage Leaves over and under them, and as much Water as will cover them, and the Bigness of a Walnut of Roche Allum: Put it on a Fire that will only keep it in a moderate Heat till it is green; then drain it off and dry it with a Cloth; put it in a Jar, and pour on it as much Vinegar boiling hot, with Cloves, Mace, Pepper and sliced Ginger, as will cover it; stop it close, if the Samphire is yellow, and has been in Pickle before, green it the same Way. Observe, that all Sorts of Spices are to be put on Pickles whole, except Nutmeg and Ginger.

To pickle Elder Flowers when they are green, and before they are blown.

LET them ly in a strong Pickle of Salt and Water two Days, then drain them, and put them in a Pan to green, with as much Water as will cover them, and two Gills of Vinegar; put them on a very slow Fire, and put green Blades over and under them; when they are green, dry them with a Cloth, then put them in a Jar, and pour on them as much boiling Vinegar, with Cloves, Mace, Pepper and Ginger in it, as will cover them: Potatoe-apples, and Nasturtian Buds are pickled the same Way.

To pickle Walnuts.

TAKE the Walnuts before the Shells are hard, and make a Pickle of Salt and Water, strong enough to bear an Egg, boil and skim it, and pour it on your Walnuts: Let them ly twenty Days, changing the Pickle every five Days, and boiling it every Time, then take them out, and wipe them with a Cloth: Boil as much white Wine Vinegar as will cover them, with Pepper, Cloves, Mace, Ginger and Nutmeg quartered,

slice

flice the Ginger, and let all the reft be whole : To a Hundred of Walnuts, put fix Spoonfuls of Muftard-feed, and fix Cloves of Garlick : When your Walnuts, Muftard, and Garlick are in the Jar, pour your Vinegar and Spice boiling hot on them; prick them full of Holes before you put them in the Salt and Water.

To pickle Walnuts green.

TAKE the largeft and cleareft you can get before the Shells are hard, pare them very thin, and as you pare them, throw them in Spring-water; put into the Water a Pound of Bay-falt; let them ly in it Twenty-four Hours, take them out and put them in a Jar, and between every Lair of Walnuts lay a Lair of Vine-leaves, and alfo at the Top and Bottom; then fill it up with cold Vinegar; let them ftand all Night, then pour the Vinegar from them into a Bell-metal Sauce-pan, with a Pound of Bay-falt, and let it boil; pour it hot on your Nuts, cover them clofs, and let them ftand a Week, pour off that Pickle, and rub them with a Piece of Flannel; then put them in the Jar with Vine-leaves as before, and boil frefh Vinegar with Cloves, Mace, Ginger, Nutmeg and Pepper; pour it boiling hot on them every Day for four Days, then put in with them a little Muftard feed, and either Garlick or Shalots.

To pickle Mufhrooms.

TAKE the fmall hard white Buttons, put them in Water, and wipe them with a Bit of clean white Flan-nel till all the Spots or black is off them, and as you wipe them throw them in clean Water; then put them in a Pan of clean cold Water, with the Bignefs of a Nut of Allum, and put them on the Fire; don't let them boil, but coming to it, take them off, and fpread them on a Cloth, and cover them with another; have ready boiled as much white Wine Vinegar as will cover them, white Pepper, Cloves, Mace, Ginger in it, they muft be all whole: Don't put on the Vinegar till cold;

put

put a little sweet Oil on the Top of the Bottle you put them in. Observe, that all the Water you put them in must be cold.

To pickle Onions.

TAKE small Onions, put them in a Pan of cold Water on the Fire, and when they are coming to boil, take them off, and take off all the brown Skins; lay them between two Cloths till cold, then put them in Bottles, and boil white Wine Vinegar, Pepper, Mace, Cloves, Ginger, and pour it on them.

To pickle red Cabbage.

CUT the Cabbage in thin Shaves; put it in a Goblet with a Gill of Vinegar, and a little Salt; put it on the Fire clofs covered, and let it ly for ten Minutes, shaking the Goblet very often; then put it in a well glazed Can, and boil as much Vinegar as will cover it, with whole Pepper, Cloves, Mace, and sliced Ginger, pour it on boiling hot; cover it clofs. It will be fit for eating in four Days.

To pickle Cucumbers, or Kidney beans.

PUT them in a strong Pickle of Salt and Water for four Days; then drain them off, and dry them in a Cloth; put them in a Brass Pan with green Cabbage-leaves under and over them, with as much Water as will cover them, and a little Bit of Roche Allum; put them on a very flow Fire, and change the Blades when they turn yellow, when they are very hot, take off the Pan till they are cold, then put it on again, put it on and off till they are green, then put them in a Cloth and dry them; boil white Wine Vinegar, whole Pepper, *Jamaica* Pepper, Cloves, and sliced Ginger, and when they are in the Jar, pour it on them boiling hot, cover them clofs. You may pickle any green Pickles the same Way.

To

To pickle Cucumbers in Slices.

CUT large green Cucumbers in Slices, not too thin, put them in a broad Pan, with some small peeled Onions; let them stand twenty four Hours close cover'd; then put them in a Sieve to drain: Boil as much Vinegar as will cover them, whole Pepper, Mace, Ginger and a little Salt; and when they are in the Jar pour it boiling hot on them: Cover them close, boil the Vinegar every Day for four or five Days, then they will be fit for Use.

To pickle Mangoes.

TAKE the largest green Cucumbers you can get, and cut a Piece out of the Side, and take out all the Seeds, fill them with Muftard, whole Pepper, Cloves, Mace and Ginger fliced; put in them Garlick or Rockambole or Shalots; then put in the Piece you cut out of the Side, and tye it faft: Green them as you do Cucumbers; dry them, put them in a Jar, pour over them Vinegar boiling hot. Let all Sorts of Spice be boil'd in it.

To pickle Colliflowers.

TAKE Colliflowers, when they are as big as an Egg, clofs and white, and juft give them a Scald in boiling Water, then fpread them on a Cloth, and cover them with it, boil the beft Vinegar with whole white Pepper, Mace and Cloves; and when they are dry put them in a Jar, and pour the Vinegar when cold on them. You may pickle white Cabbage Stalks and young Turnips the fame Way, but pare the Turnips, and cut them the Bignefs of Mushrooms.

To pickle Colliflowers red.

CUT them in small Pieces, but leave on them a fhort Stalk, put in a Chopin of Vinegar, three Pennyworth of Cochineal, a little *Jamaica* and black Pepper, and a little Salt, boil it and pour it hot over the Colliflowers: Let it ftand two or three Days close covered;

Y   fcald

scald it every three Days till it is red.   The Cochineal must be very finely pounded.

To pickle *Asparagus*.

TAKE the largest Asparagus that is very green, cut off the white, and scrape them lightly to the Head, then put them in a Jar, and throw over them some Salt, and a few Cloves and Mace, and pour on them as much Vinegar as will cover them : Let them lye nine Days, then put the Vinegar in a Brass Kettle, and put the Asparagus into it, stow them down closs, let them stand a little, then set them on the Fire until they are green ; then put them in a Jar, and tye them close.

To pickle *Plumbs* like *Olives*.

MAKE a Pickle of Water, Vinegar, white Wine and Fennel-seed, boil it, put in as much of each as will give the Pickle a Taste, then put in the Plumbs, and take them off the Fire presently.   Let them stand till they are cold, and put them in Bottles.

To pickle *Sellery*.

CUT Sellery two Inches long, put them in Salt and Water when it boils, and let them boil two or three Minutes, let them cool, and boil Vinegar, Pepper, Cloves and Ginger; and when cold, pour it on them.

To pickle *Codlins* like *Mangoes*.

GET Codlins full grown, but not full ripe, put them in Salt and Water that will bear an Egg, let them lye in it nine Days, shift the Pickles every two Days, then dry them; take out the Stalk so whole that it may fit again ; and scoop out the Core, but leave the Eye in them ; fill in the Room of the Core, with whole Mustard, a Clove of Garlick, Pepper, Mace and Cloves, Put in your Piece, and tye it up tight, boil as much Vinegar as will cover them, whole Pepper, Cloves, Mace
and

and fliced Ginger, pour it boiling hot upon them e-
very Day for a Fortnight.   Cover them clofs.

To make Goofeberry Vinegar.

BRUISE the Goofeberries with your Hand when
they are full ripe, and to every Chopin of Goofeberries, put three Chopins of Water boil'd, and let it be
put cold on them, and let it ftand twenty four Hours,
then ftrain it through Canvas or Flannel ; to four
Chopins of it put a Pound of brown Sugar, ftir it well
and put it in a Barrel , let it lye three Quarters of a
Year, but the longer the better: It is good for pickling.

Mufhroom Powder.

TAKE a Fourth part of large Mufhrooms, rub them
clean, but don't take out the Infide or Skins ; put to
them fixteen Blades of Mace, forty Cloves, a Spoonful of Pepper and a Handful of Salt, the Bignefs of
an Egg of Butter, two|Gills of Vinegar ; let all ftew faft
on the Fire, keep them ftirring till they have fpent
their Liquor; keep the Liquor for any favoury Difhes,
and dry the Mufhrooms firft on a Difh in the Oven,
then on Sieves, till they are dry enough to pound.
It will keep four or five Years, and a little of it will re-
lifh any Meat Difh.

To codle the right Codlin with Cream.

PUT the Codlins in a Stew-pan, with as much
Water as will cover them , fet them on a flow Fire till
the Skin peels off them, then take them up and peel
them ; put them in a very thin Syrup, with fome of
the Leaves of Apple Trees: Cover them clofs and put
them on the Fire again, and let them fimmer, but not
boil : When they are green and tender, clarify half a
Pound of Sugar, and boil the Codlins in it : Set them
to fimmer on a very flow Fire, then fet them to cool, and
boil half a Mutchkin of Cream ; thicken it with the Yolks
of three Eggs : Put in it two Spoonfuls of Rofe-water,

fweeten

sweeten it to your Taste, and when it is cold, pour it over the Apples.

To keep Fruit for Tarts.

PULL the Gooseberries before they are full ripe, pick off the black Eyes and the Stems; get wide mouthed Bottles, that are very dry and sweet, put your Gooseberries in them, cork the Bottles well, put them in an Oven almost cold, and let them lye in it till they turn white; then take out the Bottles, and when they are cold, rosin the Corks, and put them in a cold but not a damp Place. You may bottle red, white and black Currants, but they must be ripe.

To keep Damsons or small Plumbs for Tarts.

PUT them in a Lime-Can: To six Pounds of Damsons put three Pounds of *Lisbon* Sugar, then put coarse Paste on the Can, and put it in the Oven for an Hour, when you are going to make Use of them, take them up with a Horn or wooden Spoon: Never put your Hand in any preserved Fruit, for it will spoil them.

To make a Pupton of Apples.

PARE some Apples, take out the Cores, put them in a Sauce pan, and chop them grosly; to three Mutchkins of these Apples put in a Quarter of a Pound of Sugar, and two Spoonfuls of Water. Put them on a slow Fire, keep them stirring, grate the Rind of an Orange and Lemon in it: When it is quite thick as Marmalade, let it stand till cold, then beat up the Yolks of four Eggs, and stir in a Handful of grated Bread, and a Quarter of a Pound of sweet Butter: Mix them all together, form it into what Shape you please, and bake it in a slow Oven; then put it on a Plate upside down, for a second Course or Supper.

To make black Caps.

CUT twelve large Apples in Halves, and take out the Cores; place them on a white Iron Patty-pan with their Skins on; put to them four Spoonfuls of Rose-water, and grate fine Sugar over them; set them in a hot Oven till the Skins are black a little, and the Apples tender, so serve them up; and when you dish them, grate more Sugar over them.

To bake Apples.

PUT your Apples in an Earthen Can, with a few Cloves, a little Lemon-peel, coarse Sugar, and a Glass of red Wine, cover them close; they will take an Hour's baking in a quick Oven. You may do Pears the same Way, but they will take two Hours Baking.

To stew Apples in Halves.

PARE them, and cut them in Halves, and take out the Cores. To eight Apples, put a Chopin of Water, a Quarter of a Pound of Sugar, the Rind of a Lemon and Orange cut in small Strings; put them in a Pan, cover them, and put them over the Fire; when they are soft, serve them up with Lemon and Orange-peel about them, and the Syrup. You may do them the same Way, without taking off the Skin.

To preserve Apples for Tarts, or Torts, for a Year.

PULL the right Sort of white Codlins, when they are no bigger than large Walnuts, and some of the Leaves, put them in a Pan of cold Water, and put them on a slow Fire, when they turn white, take them up one by one, lay them on a Cloth, don't let them touch one another; cover them till both them and their Liquor is cold, then put them in a well glaz'd Can, and pour the Liquor over them; pour some render'd Sewet over them, and tye them up close with a Bladder: When you are going to use them, take off their Skin, and put them, a little of their own

Liquor,

Liquor, and a Bit of fine Loaf-sugar in a preserving Pan; cover them with Water, put green Kail Leaves over them, and set them on a slow Fire till they are green, then boil up a Syrup of fine Sugar, and put them in it, and let them simmer in it for an Hour. You may send them when cold to Table, in the Syrup, with Rose-water in it, or bake them in Tarts, or Torts.

To make a Caudle for Apple or Gooseberry Torts.

BOIL a half Mutchkin of Cream, with a Stick of Cinnamon, the Rind of a Lemon, and a little Sugar; thicken it with the Yolks of two Eggs: When your Tort is cold, and your Cream, put in it two or three Spoonfuls of Rose-water, and pour it over the Tort.

To preserve Gooseberries green.

TAKE the fairest green Gooseberries and largest, pick off the black Tops, and caudle them in fair Water, then peel them, and put them into the warm Water as you peel them: When they are all done, set them over a very slow Fire not to boil, and cover them closs till they look very clear and green, have ready some Jelly of Gooseberries made of the greenest Gaskins, boil it uncovered very fast till they are to Pieces; strain out the Jelly and the Gooseberries into it, and the same Weight of fine Sugar, boil and skim them till they are enough, then glass them up.

To preserve Pears

TAKE the best preserving Pears fresh pulled, make a small Hole at the black End, and pick out the Seeds with a Needle-head, then put them in scalding Water, and take the Skin off them, then take their equal Weight of fine Sugar, and take the same Water your Pears were boiled in, and mix the Sugar with as much of the Water as will cover the Pears; then let it come a-boiling, and skim it; put in your Pears, and let them boil till they be soft, then take them out, and boil up

your

your Syrup, and when they are both cold, lay in your Pears in Gally pots; pour the Syrup over them before you boil them, put a Clove in every Hole, pour Jelly of Apples over them, and they will keep a great while.

To preserve Raspberries whole

TAKE the faireſt and largeſt Raſpberries you can get, and to every Pound of Raſps, add a Pound and a half of fine Sugar; clarify it and boil it till it blows very ſtrong, put in the Raſps, and let them boil as quick as poſſible, ſtrewing ſome fine beat Sugar on them as they boil: When the Sugar boils over them, take them off, and let them ſtand to cool, then put them on the Fire again; put to every Pound of Raſps two Gills of Currant Jelly; then boil it till the Syrup hangs in Flax from the Spoon, keep them well ſkimmed, then put them in Glaſſes when they are almoſt cold.

To make Raspberry Jam.

PICK them clean, and to every Pound of Raſps put two Gills of Currant Juice, and a Pound and a half of Sugar, boil them on a quick Fire, and when they fall to the Bottom, they are enough.

To preserve the green admirable Plumb.

TAKE theſe Plumbs when full grown, and juſt on the Turn; prick them with a large Needle, and ſet them on the Fire with as much Water as will cover them, with green Kail-leaves under and over them; let them green very gradually, they muſt not boil; then drain them, and boil them in clarified Sugar, let them cool a little, and give them another Boil if they ſhrink, prick them with a Fork in the Syrup, and give them another Boil; put a Sheet of clean white Paper over them, and ſet them by; next Day boil ſome Sugar till it blows, and put it to them, and give them a good Boil, then put them by for Uſe.

To preserve Gooseberries whole.

TAKE the largest preserving Gooseberries, and pick off the black Eye, but not the Stalk; set them over the Fire in a Pot of Water to scald, cover them very closs, and let them scald, but not boil, or break, and when they are tender, take them up in cold Water; then take a Pound and a Half of double refined Sugar to a Pound of Gooseberries; clarify the Sugar with Water, and when the Syrup is cold, put your Gooseberries into your preserving Pan, and put the Syrup to them; set them on a gentle Fire, and let them boil, but not too fast, lest they break; when you perceive the Sugar has entered them, take them off, cover them with white Pepper, and set them by till the next Day, then take them out of the Syrup, and boil the Syrup till it begins to rope, skim it and put it to them again, and set them on a gentle Fire till you perceive the Syrup will rope; then take them off, and when cold cover them with Paper; boil some Gooseberries to Jelly, and put them in Glasses, and cover them with it.

To scald Fruit for present Use:

PUT your Fruit in boiling Water, as much as will cover them; set them on a slow Fire till they are tender, turning them often, lay a Paper closs on them; let them stand till cold. To a Pound of Fruit put half a Pound of Sugar, let it boil, but not fast, till it looks clear: If you do whole Pipins, you must cut Orange and Lemon-peel as small as Straw, and put them and the Juice of Lemon in them.

To make white Quince Marmalade.

SCALD your Quinces tender, take off the Skin, and pulp them from the Core very fine,: To every Pound of Quinces put a Pound and a half of fine Sugar in Lumps, and two Gills of Water, dip your Sugar in Water, and boil and skim it till it is a thick
Syrup

Syrup, then put in your Quinces. Boil it on a quick Fire.

To preserve Apricocks.

PULL the fairest Apricocks before they are too ripe, wipe them, and put them in a Pan of cold Water, set them on the Fire, and when the Water is just scalding hot, take them off and skin them, and as you skin them, grate Sugar on them : If there are any Bits that want Skin pare it off very thin with a Pen-knife ; then take out the Stones on the Side that has a Crefs in it, but don't break the Apricock : If there are any very hard to come out, let them alone till they are boiled in the Syrup. To every Pound of them put a Pound of very fine Loaf sugar ; dip it in Water, and boil it ; skim it, and then put in the Apricocks ; let them ly in it till the Syrup is cold, then put them on a slow Fire, and let them simmer, cover them with a clean Sheet of Paper , take them off again, and let them cool ; break the Stones, and take out your Kernels whole, put them in with the Apricocks ; put them on and off the Fire three or four Times, still letting them cool till the Syrup penetrates into them, then let them boil till they are clear, take care they don't break ; never let them boil till the last Time, only simmer ; then put them in Gallypots, and when cold, paper them. Take the Skins off the Kernels.

To preserve red or white Currants whole.

PULL the largest Branches and biggest Kernels you can get ; make a very small Slit in the Side of them with a Needle, and pick out the Seeds ; hold them very gently in your Fingers, for Fear of bruising or pulling them off the Stems : To every Pound of Currants, you must have two Pounds of clarified double refined Sugar, and put the Currants in it on a clear Fire : The red must have half a Mutchkin of the Juice of red Currants in it, and you must boil both till they are quite clear on a quick Fire.

Z

To preferve Pears red.

TAKE the large Pound Pears, when full ripe, pare them, and put them in as much Water as will cover them, then put in a Penny-worth of pounded Cochi neal, and let them boil till they are tender ; then put in the Weight of your Pears of Sugar, and let it boil to a thick Syrup , cover your Pears till you boil and fkim your Syrup , then put in your Pears, and let them boil till they are red and clear : put the Rind of a Le mon and Orange cut in Strings, and fqueeze in the Juice in the Syrup before it comes to boil : Put them in Gallypots, and put on them the Jelly of red Goofe-berries, it is made as the Jelly of green Goofeberries.

To make Marmalade of Oranges.

TAKE your Oranges, grate them, cut them in Quarters, take the Skins off them, and take the Pulp from the Strings and Seeds ; put the Skins in a Pan of Spring-water, boil them till they are very tender, then take them out of the Water, and cut them in very thin Slices ; beat fome in a Marble Mortar, and leave the thin Slices to boil by themfelves. To every Pound of Oranges put a Pound of fine Sugar , firft wet the Sugar in Water, boil it a good while, then put in Half of the Pulp, keep the other Half for the fliced Oranges, to every Mutchkin of the Pulp you muft put in a Pound of Sugar likeways, then put in the grated Rind, boil it till it is very clear, then put it in Gallypots , when cold, paper them.   Boil your Chips the fame Way, but don't mix the pounded with them.

To preferve Goofeberries for Tarts.

PICK them clean, and to every ten Pounds of Goofe-berries put eight Pounds of fine powdered Sugar, and two Gills of Water , put them on a flow Fire till the Sugar is well fimmered among them , fkim them, and then let them boil as faft as you pleafe : Boil them till they are very clear, and will jelly. You may preferve
greer

green Gaskens, and red and white Goofeberries for Tarts, the fame Way.

To preferve white Plumbs.

TAKE your Plumbs before they are too ripe, give them a Slit in the Seam, and prick them behind, make your Water almoft fcalding hot, and put a little Sugar into it, and put in your Plumbs, and cover them clofs, fet them on the Fire to coddle, and take them off a little and fet them on again, take care they do not break, boil to a Height as much refined Sugar as will cover them, and when they are coddled pretty tender, take them out of the Liquor, and put them into your preferving Pan to your Syrup, which muft be Blood warm: Let them boil till they are clear, fkim them, and take them off, and let them ftand two Hours, then fet them on, and boil them again, when they are clear put them in Glaffes, boil your Syrup till it is thick, and when cold pour it on your Plumbs. Put Jelly of Pipins over them.

To preferve Damfons.

TAKE fome Damfons, and cut them in Pieces, and put them in a Skellet over the Fire, with as much Water as will cover them; when they boil, and the Liquor pretty ftrong, ftrain it out: Add for every Pound of your whole Damfons a Pound of double refined Sugar, put the third Part of the Sugar in the Liquor, and fet it on the Fire, and when it fimmers put in your whole Damfons, wipe them clean, let them have one good Boil, take them off for half an Hour, and cover them up clofs, then fet them on again, and let them fimmer over the Fire, often turning them: Take them out, and put them in a Bafon, and ftrew all the Sugar you left on them, and pour the hot Liquor over them, and cover them up, and let them ftand till next Day; then boil them up again till they are e-nough, take them up and put them in Pots, boil the
Liquor

Liquor till it jellies, and pour it on them when it is almoft cold, fo paper them.

To preferve green Plumbs.

TAKE green Plumbs before they begin to ripen, let them be carefully gathered, with their Stalks and Leaves, put them in cold Spring-water over a Fire, and let them boil very gently ; when they will peel take off the Skins, and put the Plumbs in other cold Water, and let them ftand over a very gentle Fire till they are foft, put two Pounds of double refined Sugar to every Pound of Plumbs, and make the Sugar with fome Water into a very thick Syrup. Before the Plumbs are put in it, the Stones of the Plumbs muft be as foft as you may thruft a Pin in them.   After the fame Manner do green Apricocks.

To preferve Mulberries.

SET fome Mulberries on the Fire, and draw from them a Mutchkin of Juice, put to it three Pounds of Sugar, boil your Syrup and skim it, and put into it two Pounds of ripe Mulberries, and let them ftand in the Syrup till they are thoroughly warm, then fet them on the Fire, and let them boil gently, then put them by till next Day, then boil them ; and when the Syrup is pretty thick, and the Drop ftands, they are enough, fo put them in Glaffes, and paper them when cold.

Jelly of Goofeberries.

TAKE your Goofeberries when they are at full Growth, but not ripe, fill a Pint ftoup, and ftop the Mouth of it, and put it in a Pot of Water, and let it boil till they are tender; then put them in a Search, and let the Juice drain from them, then fill up the Stoup again, and do fo till you have ftewed all you have a mind to do, to every Mutchkin of Juice put a Pound and a Quarter of fine Sugar, and when diffolved, boil it as you did the Apple Jelly.

To

To preserve golden Pipins red.

PARE them, and make a Hole in them through the Heart with a Skewer; put them in a Pan with as much Water as will cover them; put a Penny-worth of Cochineal in a Bit of Muslin, and put it in; cut the Rind of a Lemon or Orange in long small Strings, and put that and the Juice in them, let them simmer till they are a little tender, then put in two Pounds of fine Loaf-sugar to a Dozen, and let it dissolve, then put them on a quick Fire, and let them boil very fast till they are a clear red, and very tender; the faster they boil, the wholler they will be. You must not cover them at all, but stand and keep them under the Syrup with a Silver-spoon, they take a long Time to boil. You may do them clear the same Way, leaving out the Cochineal. A Bath-metal Skellet is the best to do them in.

To make Marmalade of Plumbs or any Fruit.

PUT them in a Stoup, and put the Stoup in a Pot of Water; let it stew till they are very tender, then rub them through a Search; put to them their equal Weight of fine Sugar, and boil them to a Marmalade; break the Sugar very small before you put it in the Marmalade.

To make a Syrup of Nettles.

PICK the young red Nettles in *April*, and put them in a Pint stoup, put the Stoup in a Pot of Water, and let them simmer for twelve Hours, then squeeze out the Tincture, and put it in a clean Pan, beat the Whites of two Eggs and mix with it, and when it boils, skim it, and to every Mutchkin of Tincture put a Pound of brown Sugar-candy: When it is dissolved, set it on the Fire, and boil it up to a Syrup, then let it cool, and bottle it, put no Water to the Nettles.——They are good for Consumptions.

Syrup

Syrup of Maiden-hair.

FILL a Pint Stoup as much as it will hold, and put as much Water as will cover it, and set it on the Side of the Fire, and let it stand twenty four Hours, then try if all the Taste be from it, if not, set it nearer the Fire, and let it boil, then strain it, and to every Mutchkin of the Tincture put a Pound of white Sugar-candy, and two Drops of Cinnamon, and a Drop of Mace, they must be whole, boil all together to a Syrup, and when cold bottle it. You may make any Herb syrup the same Way.

To make Jelly of Apples the Colour of Amber.

TAKE big Pipins, pare them and take out the Cores, and boil them in a Chopin of Water till it comes to a Mutchkin; put in it two Spoonfuls of Rose water, a Pound of fine Sugar, boil it uncovered till it comes to the right Colour; drop a little on a Piece of Glass, and if it stands upright, it is enough, put it in Glasses or Gallypots. You may make red Jelly the same Way, but colour the Water with a little Cochineal.

Gooseberry Jam.

TAKE the green Gooseberries full ripe, top and tail them, and weigh them, put a Pound of Fruit to three Quarters of a Pound of fine Sugar, and two Gills of Water; boil the Sugar and Water together, skim it and put in your Gooseberries, and boil them till they are clear and tender, then put them in Pots.

To preserve Cherries.

TAKE the best Morello Cherries when full ripe, either stone them, or clip off Part of the Stalks; to every Pound take a Pound of Sugar, and boil it till it blows very strong, then put in your Cherries, and by Degrees bring them to boil as fast as you can, that the Sugar may come over them; skim them, and set them by, next Day boil a Mutchkin of the Juice of
red

red Currants, and a Pound of Sugar, and skim it, and put it in the Cherries, then give all a Boil together: When almoft cold, place them in Glaffes, and pour the Syrup on them.

To make Currant Jelly.

MASH the Currants, and put them on the Fire, then fqueeze out all the Juice, and to every *English* Quart, put two Pounds of Sugar, put it on the Fire and boil it, keep it well fkimmed, and ftir it till the Sugar diffolves: When it boils twelve Minutes, drop a little on a Plate, and if it jellies, take it off and put it in Glaffes, the finer the Sugar is, the better for all Sweet-meats· If it is white Currants, clarify the Sugar, and ftrain the Juice.

To make Conferve of Rofes.

TAKE the Scarlet Buds before they are ripe, and cut off all the Whites, then weigh all the Rofes, and put them into a Mortar, and beat them extraordinary well, till they be like Powder, then take the triple Weight of your Rofes in Sugar, well fearched, and put it in by Degrees, always beating them, and as it diffolves, put in more, till your Sugar be all made Ufe of, and when it is all well mixed, put it up in your Gallypots, and fet it againft the Sun, ftir them once in two or three Days for a Fortnight, then it is fit for Ufe: After this Manner you may make Conferve of Violets or Gilliflowers.

Clear Pipin Jelly.

TAKE fourteen good Pipins, and throw them into cold Water; fet them on the Fire till they are diffolved, then ftrain them, and to a Mutchkin of it put a Pound of double refined Sugar; let it boil very faft, and keep it clean fkimmed, then put in it the Juice of two large Lemons: As it is boiling, try it on a Plate,
and

and when you find it jellies, it is enough. You may put a Chopin of Water in it.

Jelly of Pipins with Slices.

BOIL a Mutchkin of Water and a Pound of Sugar, with fix Pipins, the Juice of a Lemon and Orange, to a clear Jelly; then pare and core three Pipins, and cut them in Slices, and put them in your Jelly, and boil them very quick, till they are clear, but don't let them break, fo put them in Glaffes.

To colour Jellies.

JELLIES made of Hartſhorn or Calves Feet, may be made of what Colour you pleaſe. If white, uſe Almonds pounded and ſtrained after the uſual Manner, if yellow, put in Yolks of Eggs, or a little Saffron ſteeped and ſqueezed, if red, ſome Juice of Beet-root or Cochineal; if purple, Turnſole or Powder of Violets; if green, Juice of Beets or Spinage.

A very fine Way to dry Cherries.

TO every five Pound of ſton'd Cherries, take a Pound of double refined Sugar, put the Cherries into the preſerving Pan, with a very little Water: Make both but juſt ſcalding hot, take them immediately out of this Liquor, and dry them, then put them again into the Pan, and ſtrew on Sugar between every Lair of Cherries; let it ſtand to melt, and then ſet it on the Fire, and make it ſcalding hot, as before, which muſt be done twice or thrice with the Sugar, then drain them from the Syrup, and lay them fing-ly to dry in the Sun, or in the Stove. When they are dry, throw them into a Baſon of cold Water, and take them immediately out, and dry them with a Cloth; ſet them again in the hot Sun, or in the Stove, and keep them in a dry Place all the Year. This is
not

not only the beſl Way to give them a good Taſte, but alſo the moſt certain Way for Colour and Plumpneſs.

Currants preſerved in Bunches.

STONE your Currants, and tye them up in ſmall Bunches: To every Pound of Currants, boil two Pounds of Sugar, till it blows very ſtrong; then ſlip in the Currants, and give them a quick Boil, till the Sugar covers them; let them ſettle a Quarter of an Hour, then let them boil till the Sugar riſes almoſt to the Top of the Pan; then let them ſettle, ſkim them, and ſet them by till next Day, then drain them and lay them out, taking Care to ſpread out the Sprigs, that they may not ſtick together; then duſt them well, and dry them in a hot Stove.

Currants in Jelly.

STRIP the Currants, and put them in an earthen Pot, tye them cloſs down, and ſet them in a Kettle of boiling Water, and let them ſtand three Hours, the Kettle ſtill boiling; then take a clean flaxen Cloth, and ſtrain out the Juice, and when it is ſettled, take a Pound of double refined Sugar beaten and ſifted, and put to it a Mutchkin of clear Juice: Have ready ſome whole Currants ſton'd, and put them in when the Juice boils, and let them boil till the Syrup jellies, which you may know by trying it in a Spoon, then put it in Glaſſes. Make Jelly of Currants the ſame Way, only leave out the whole Currants. When cold, paper them up.

To preſerve Raſpberries liquid.

TAKE the faireſt and largeſt Raſpberries you can get, and to every Pound of Raſps, take a Pound and a half of Sugar, clarify it, and boil it till it blows very ſtrong: Put in the Raſps, and let them boil as quick as poſſible, ſtrewing ſome fine beat Sugar on them as they boil: When they have had a good Boil, and that the Sugar riſes all over them, take them off and let

A a   them

them settle a little ; then give them another Boil, and
put to every Pound of Rasps half a Pint of Currant
Jelly ; give them a good Boil, till you perceive the
Syrup hangs in Flaiks from your Skimmer, then take
them from the Fire, take off the Scum, and put them
into Glasses or Pots. Take the Scum clean off the
Top ; when cold, make a Jelly of Currants, and fill
up your Glasses ; cover them with Paper, first wet in
Water, and dried a little betwixt two Cloths, which
Paper you must put close to the Jelly, then wipe the
Glasses clean, and cover the Tops with the dry Paper.

Raspberry Cakes.

PICK away all the Stems and spotted Raspberries,
then bruise the rest through a Hair-sieve into an earthen Pan, and put on a Board or Weight to press out
all the Water you can ; then pour the Paste into the
Preserving-pan, and dry it over the Fire till there is no
Moisture in it, that is, no Juice that will run from it,
stirring it closs to keep it from burning : To every
Pound take a Pound and two Ounces of Sugar finely
beat, and put it in gradually : When all is in put it
on the Fire, and let it incorporate well together ; then
take it off and scrape it all to one Side of the Pan,
let it cool a very little, and put it into Moulds ; when
quite cold, put them into the Stove without dusting,
and dry it as other Paste. Take Care the Paste does
not boil after the Sugar is in, for it will make it grea-
sy, and hinder it to dry.

Raspberry clear Cakes:

TAKE two Quarts of ripe Gooseberries, and a
Quart of red Raspberries, put them into a Stone Jug,
and stop them closs, then set them into a Pot of
cold Water, as much as covers the Neck of the Jug,
and let it boil till it comes to a Paste, then put them
into a Hair-sieve, and press out all the Jelly into a
Pan, and strain it through a Jelly-bag. To every Pound
                                                     put

put twenty Ounces of double refined Sugar, and boil it till it crack in the Water; then take it off, and put in the Jelly, and stir it over a slow Fire till all the Sugar is melted; then give it a good Fleet till it is well incorporated; then take it off and skim it well, and fill your clear Cake Glasses; take off the Skim, and put it into the Stove to dry. When they begin to crust on the upper Side, turn them out upon square Glasses, and set them to dry again. When they begin to have a tender Candy, cut them into Quarters, or as you please, and set them to dry till hard; then turn them on Sieves, and when thoroughly dry, put them into Boxes. In filling up your clear Cakes and clear Paste, you must be as expeditious as possible, for if it cools, it will be a Jelly before you can get it in. White Raspberry clear Cakes are made the same Way, only mixing them with the Gooseberries in the Infusion.

To preserve green Amber Plumbs.

TAKE green Amber Plumbs when full grown, prick them in two or three Places, and put them in cold Water, set them over the Fire to scald, and take care not to let the Water become too hot, lest it spoil them: When they are very tender, put them into a very thin Sugar, that is to say, one Part Sugar and two Parts Water, give them a little Warm in it, and set them by covered: Next Day give them another Warm, and the third Day drain them, and boil up the Syrup, adding a little more Sugar, then put the Syrup to the Plumbs, and give them a Warm. Next Day do the same, the Day following boil the Syrup till it is a little smooth, put in the Plumbs, and give them a Boil, the next Day boil the Syrup till very smooth, put it to the Plumbs and cover them, and put them in the Stove; next Day boil some Sugar to blow very strong, put it to the Fruit, and give all a Boil, then put it into the Stove for two Days, then drain them and lay them
out

out to dry; firſt duſting them very well, and manage them in the drying as any other Fruit.

To preſerve the green *Mogul Plumb.*

• LET it be juſt upon the turning ripe, prick it into the Stone on that Side where the Clift is with a Pen-knife, and as you do them throw them into cold Water, and ſet them over a very ſlow Fire to ſcald, when they are very tender take them carefully out of the Water, and put them into a thin Sugar, half Sugar, half Water, warm them gently, cover them and ſet them by: The next Day drain off the Syrup and boil it ſmooth, adding a little freſh Sugar, and give them a gentle Boil; the Day following boil the Sugar very ſmooth, and pour it on them, and ſet them in the Stove for two Days, then drain them, and boil freſh Sugar very ſmooth, juſt to blow a little, put in your Plumbs, and give them a good covered Boil-ing, ſkim them and put them into the Stove for two Days, drain them and lay them out to dry, duſting them very well.

To preſerve yellow *Amber Plumbs.*

TAKE them when full ripe, put them into the preſerving Pan with as much Sugar as will cover them, and give them a good Boil; let them ſettle a little, and give them another Boil three or four Times round the Fire, ſkim them, and next Day drain off the Sy-rup; put them again into the Pan, and boil as much freſh Sugar as will cover them to blow. Give them a thorough Boiling, and ſkim them, and ſet them in the Stove twenty four Hours; then drain them, and lay them out to dry. Duſt them firſt.

To preſerve green *Grapes.*

TAKE the largeſt and fineſt Grapes before they are thorough ripe, ſtone them and ſcald them, and let them ly two Days in the Water they are ſcalded in,
then

then drain them and put them into a thin Syrup, and give them a Heat over a flow Fire : Next Day turn them in the Pan, and warm them again : Next Day drain them, and give them a good Boil in clarified Sugar, and skim them and set them by : The Day following boil some Sugar to blow, and put in the Grapes, and give them a good Boil ; skim them, and set them in a warm Stove all Night ; drain them next Day, and lay them out to dry, having dusted them well.

Green Apricocks.

TAKE them before the Stones are hard, wet them and lay them in a coarse Cloth with two or three Handfuls of Salt, and rub them till the Roughness is off ; then put them in scalding Water, and let them be almost boiled ; then set them off till almost cold, do this two or three Times : After this let them be closs covered, and when they look green, let them boil till they begin to be tender, take their Weight of double refined Sugar, and to a Pound of Sugar two Gills of Water ; make the Syrup, and when it is almost cold, put in the Apricocks, boil them till they are clear ; warm your Syrup three or four Times till it is thick. You may put them in cold Jelly, or dry them as you use them.

Apricock Chips.

SLICE the Apricocks the long Way, but not pare them ; take their Weight of double refined Sugar, boil it to a thin Candy, put in the Apricocks, and let them stand on the Fire till they are scalding hot ; let them ly a Night in the Liquor, then lay them on thin Plates, and set them in the Sun to dry.

Jam Apricocks.

PARE them and take out the Stones, break them and take out the Kernels, and blanch them, to every Pound of Apricocks boil a Pound of Sugar till it blows very strong, put in the Apricocks and give them a
quick

quick Boil till they are broke, then take them off and bruife them well, put in the Kernels and ftir all together on the Fire, and fill your Pots or Glaffes with them. If it is too fweet, fharpen it with a little white Currant Jelly to your Tafte.

To preferve green Walnuts.

GATHER them in fair Weather, and before the Shell grows hard; boil them in Water to take off the Bitternefs, then put them into cold Water, peel off the Rind, and lay them in a Pan with a Lair of Sugar equal to the Weight of the Nuts, and as much Water as will wet it. When they are boiled up over a moderate Fire and cooled, do the fame Thing again, and fet them by for Ufe.

To preferve Mulberries liquid.

TAKE two Quarts of Mulberry Juice, ftrain it, boil it over a gentle Fire, with a Pound and a half of Sugar till it become a Kind of Syrup; then flip into the Pan three Quarts of Mulberries not over ripe: Give them a Boil, then pour all into an Earthen Veffel, ftop it clofs, and keep it for Ufe.

Another Way.

BOIL the Sugar till a little pearled, allowing three Pounds to four Pounds of Mulberries, and give them a light covered Boiling in the fame Sugar, fhaking the Pan gently, then fet it by till next Day, then drain off the Syrup in order to bring it to its pearled Quality, then flip in the Fruit, adding a little more pearled Sugar if needful: When cold enough, put it into Pots.

To preferve Seville Oranges in Quarters, or in Sticks.

EITHER zeaft or turn your Oranges according as you defign to do them, whether in Zeafts, Chips or Faggots. *Turning,* in this Senfe, is a Term of Art which denotes a particular Manner of paring Oranges and

and Lemons, when the outer Rind or Peel is pared off very thin and narrow with a Knife for the Purpose, winding it about the Fruit, so as the Peel may extend to a very great Length without breaking. To *zeaſt,* is to cut the Peel from Top to Bottom in ſmall Slips as thin as poſſible. The Orange thus prepared may be cut into Quarters, or into Sticks as you pleaſe. You muſt take away the inſide Skin and the Juice; ſet them over the Fire in Water, do not put them in till the Water begins to boil, and when they are done enough, (which you will know by their ſlipping of a Pin when ſtuck into them) let them cool, and put them into freſh Water, and next into clarified Sugar, let them have ſeven or eight covered Boilings before you ſet them by to cool. Boil them over again till the Syrup is almoſt ſmooth; drain them next Day and put them into Pots, let your Syrup be pearled, and pour it on them. Keep them in that Way till you think fit to dry them.

Oranges preſerved in Slips.

WHEN the Fruit is zeaſted, cut the Pulp into Slips, which are to be ſlit again in their Thickneſs to make them very thin, ſcald theſe Slips in Water till they are very ſoft, then throw them into clarified Sugar newly paſſed thro' the ſtraining Bag when it is ready to boil, and give it twenty Boilings: Next Day having brought your Sugar to the ſmooth Quality, put the Slips into it, and give them ſeven or eight Boilings: The third Day boil your Sugar till pearled, and give them a covered Boiling. Some Time after put them into Pots, and you may dry them as Occaſion ſerves. Lemons, Limes and Citrons are preſerved much the ſame Way, either intire, or in Sticks, Faggots, Zeaſts, Slips, &c.

Red criſp Almonds, or Prawlings.

MELT a Pound of Loaf or powdered Sugar with a little Water, and let a Pound of Almonds be boiled

in

in it till they crackle; add as much Cochineal as will give it a right red, let it boil again to its cracked Quality, and at that inftant tofs in your Almonds; and removing the Pan from the Fire, ftir them clofs till they are dry.   The Cochineal may be prepared by boiling it with Allum and Cream of Tartar, which Liquor is generally ufed for every Thing that is to be brought to a fine Colour, as Marmalades, Jellies, Paftes, Creams, &c.

To preferve white Citrons.

CUT them in Pieces of what Size you pleafe, put them in Salt and Water for four or five Hours; wafh them and boil them tender, then drain them and put them into as much clarified Sugar as will cover them, and fet them by till next Day; drain them and boil the Syrup a little fmooth, when cool, put it on the Citrons; next Day boil your Syrup quite fmooth, and pour it on the Citrons; the Day after boil all together, and put it into a Pot to be candied, or put in Jelly or Compofts as you pleafe.   You muft look over thefe Fruits fo kept in Syrup, and if you perceive any Froth on them, give them a Boil, and if they fhould become very frothy and four, boil firft the Syrup, and then all together.

To make clear Quince Cakes.

BOIL and clarify over a Fire a Pint of the Syrup of Quinces, with a Quart or two of Rafpberries, fkim it well from Time to Time, add a Pound and a half of Sugar, and boil up the fame Quantity of Sugar to a Candy Height, and pour it in hot; ftir all together, and keep it clofs ftirring till it is almoft cold, then fpread it upon Plates, and cut it into Cakes of what Shape you pleafe.

Marmalade of Apricocks.

TAKE full ripe Apricocks, pare and quarter them, and take out the Strings, put three Quarters of a Pound of Loaf Sugar to every Pound of Apricocks, and

put

put them into a pretty broad Pan; fet the Apricocks on the Fire without either Water or Sugar, keep them ftirring that they may not burn: When they are melt-ed and boiled a pretty while, ftrew in the Sugar as quick as you can, and let them boil quick till the Sy-rup is thick, and they look clear, then put them in Pots or Glaffes.

Marmalade of Apples.

SCALD them in Water, and when tender take them out and drain them. and ftrain them through a Sieve; boil your Sugar till it is well feathered, allowing three Quarters of a Pound of Sugar to every Pound of Ap-ples; temper and dry the whole over the Fire as ufu-al, and let then fimmer together; ftrew it over with fine Sugar, and put it into Pots or Glaffes.

Marmalade of Rafpberries.

MAKE the Body of this Marmalade of very ripe Currants, to which add a Handful of Rafpberries, that it may look as it were all of Rafpberries.

Marmalade of Quinces, after the Italian Manner.

PARE about thirty Quinces as thin as poffible, and take out the Cores, and put them into a Quart of Wa-ter with two Pounds of Sugar, let all boil together till they are foft; then ftrain the Juice and Pulp, and put to it four Pounds of Sugar, and boil it up to a right Confiftence.

To make Quiddany of Pipins, of an Amber or Ruby Colour.

PARE the Pipins, and cut them into Quarters, and boil them in as much Water as will cover them, till they are foft, and fink in the Water, then ftrain the Pulp. Take a Pint of the Liquor, and boil it with half a Pound of Sugar, till it appears a quaking Jelly on the Moulds. When the Quiddany is cold, turn it on a wet Trencher,

B b and

and flide it into Boxes. If you would have it of
red Colour, let it boil leifurely, clofs covered, till i
is red like Claret.

Quiddany of all Sorts of Plumbs.

BOIL the Plumbs in Apple Water till they are red
as Claret, when you have made the Liquor ftrong of
the Fruit, put to every Mutchkin half a Pound of Sugar
and let it boil till a Drop of it will hang on the Back of
a Spoon like a quaking Jelly. If you would have i
of an Amber Colour, you muft boil it on a quick Fire

Pafte of ripe Apricocks.

APRICOCK Pafte is made the fame Way as the
Marmalade, or you may fcald the Apricocks withou
Sugar, but if they are not thoroughly ripe, bruife then
well, or pound them in a Mortar. Then flip in th
Fruit into an equal Quantity of cracked Sugar, and in
corporated with it, when well dried over the Fire
then let all fimmer, and drefs your Pafte as ufual
You may dry it at the fame Time if you pleafe.

Goofeberry Pafte.

TAKE them when full grown, wafh them and pu
them into the preferving Pan, with as much Water a
covers them; boil them very thick all to a Pommifh
then ftrain them through a Hair Sieve into a Pan, and
prefs out all the Juice; and to every Pound of this Paft
take one Pound and two Ounces of Sugar, boil it til
it cracks; then mix in your Pafte, and let it incorporat
with Sugar over a flow Fire: When it is well incor
porate, fkim it, and fill your Pots, then fkim it again
and when cold put it into the Stove. When it is crufte
on the Top, turn them and fet them in the Stove again
and when a little dry cut them in long Pieces, and fe
them to dry quite. and when they are fo crufted as to
bear touching, turn them on Sieves, and dry the othe
Side, and put them into Boxes. You may make them
re

red or green, by putting the Colour, when the Sugar and Paſte is all mixed, giving it a Warm all together.

To make Ketchup.

GET the largeſt Muſhrooms, wipe them clean, and maſh them with your Hand, ſtrew on them a Handful of Salt; let them lye all Night, then put them on the Fire ten Minutes, keep them ſtirring all the while, then ſqueeze them through a Canvas, and let them ſettle; pour it from the Sediment, then put it on the Fire, and clarify it with the Whites of two Eggs; then put in it whole Pepper, Cloves, Mace, Ginger and *Jamaica* Pepper, and Salt; it muſt be very high ſeaſoned: Boil one Part of it away, and when cold bottle it, putting the Spices in the Bottles with it.

To keep Artichoke Bottoms the whole Year.

PUT them in a Pot, and put as much Water about them as will cover them, ſalt them, let them boil till the Leaves come eaſily from them; then take off every Thing of the Bottoms; put them in a ſlow Oven on or before the Fire, keep them in a dry Place, when they are thoroughly dry.

Syrup of Lemons and Oranges.

TO a Mutchkin of Juice put a Pound and a Half of fine Loaf Sugar; put it on the Fire and let it ſimmer, ſkim it and ſtir it often, then let it ſettle, and when 't is cold bottle it, but don't put the Sediment in it.

To preſerve whole Oranges.

GRATE off the Rind very gently, cut a Bit out of the Top where the Stem is, and ſcoop out all that is in them, put them in a very clean Kettle of cold Water, cover it cloſs, boil them as tender that you may thruſt a Straw in them, ſhifting the Water three or four Times, then put them between two Cloths to drain, and to every Pound of them put two Pounds of Loaf Sugar,

Sugar, with two Gills of Water, and boil it till it blows; fkim it clean; then put in the Oranges, and boil them till they are very clear, keeping them down in the Syrup with a Spoon while they are boiling: Then put them in Cans.

To preferve Angelica.

BOIL the Stalks of Angelica in Water till they are very tender, then peel them and put them into other warm Water, and cover them till they are green'd on a gentle Fire: When they are green lay them on a Cloth to dry, and take their Weight of fine Sugar, and boil it to a Syrup; tye up the Stalks in any Shape you pleafe, and boil them in the Syrup very quick; if you dry them, you muft fhake Sugar on them, and put them in a flow Oven.

To preferve Peaches in Brandy.

PUT your Peaches in boiling Water, but don't let them boil, take them out and put them in Water, dry them between two Cloths, then put them in wide mouth'd Bottles, to fix Peaches put a Quarter of a Pound of Sugar, clarify it, and put it on the Peaches, then fill up the Bottles with Brandy, ftop them clofs, and keep them in a cold Place

To dry Pears or Apples.

TAKE preferving Pears, and thruft a wooden Skewer into the Head of them beyond the Core, then pare them the long Way, and fcald them, but not too tender, then take their Weight of Sugar, and to every Pound of Sugar put two Gills of Water; clarify it, and put in your Pears, fet them on the Fire, and let them boil very quick half an Hour, cover them with white Paper, and fet them by till next Day. Then take them out of the Syrup, and boil it till it is thick and ropy, then put in the Pears, and put it on the Fire, and let the Syrup boil very faft over them · Then cover them with Paper, and fet them in the Oven, or

Stove

Stove for twenty four Hours; then take it out, and put them on a Sieve; then lay them on White-iron Plates, and duft them with fine Sugar, then put them in the Oven; and when one Side is dry lay them on Papers, and turn them, and duft the other with Sugar; fqueeze the Pears by Degrees. If you do Apples, fqueeze the Eyes to the Stalks. When they are dry put them in Boxes, with Papers between. You may do Apricocks, Peaches and Nectarines the fame Way, but when they are fcalded take out the Stones.

CHAP. VI.

Of *WINES*, &c.

To make Orange Wine.

TO fix Gallons of Water, put twelve Pounds of fingle refined Sugar, the Whites of four Eggs well beaten, put them in the cold Water; then let it boil three Quarters of an Hour, taking off the Scum as it rifes, whe it is cold put in two Spoonfuls of Barm and fix Ounces of Syrup of Lemons beaten together; put in alfo the Juice and Rinds of fifty Oranges thin pared, that no white Part, or any of the Seeds go in with the Juice which fhould be ftrained: Let all ftand two Days in an open Veffel, or large Pan, then put it in a clofs Veffel, and in three or four Days ftop it down. When it has ftood three Weeks then draw it off into another Veffel, and add to it two Quarts of Rhenifh or white Wine. Then ftop it clofs again, and in fix Weeks it will be fine to bottle, and to drink in a Month after. Obferve that an *Englifh* Gallon is two *Scots* Pints, and if the Barm be not very good, to put in thirteen or fourteen Spoonfuls.

To make Raisin Wine.

TO each five Pounds of Raisins picked clean from the Stalks, take one *English* Gallon of cold Water, chop the Raisins small, and put them into a Vessel, fit for the Quantity, then pour on the cold Water, stir them about, and cover the Vessel with a Cloth, so let them stand ten Days, stirring them about twice a-day: at the End of ten Days, strain out the Liquor through a Search, squeezing the Raisins very well, then put the Liquor into a Barrel that will just hold the Quantity you make. After a hissing Noise, which is commonly about three Weeks after, bung up the Barrel, and let it stand a Year, then bottle it for Use.

To make Vinegar.

TAKE half the Quantity of the above Water, let it be boiling hot, and pour it upon the Raisins: After you have squeezed them out of the first Liquor, and after standing, (till it is as cold as Wort, when Barm is put to it) take a Mutchkin of good Barm and put to it, and let it work two Weeks, stirring it once or twice a-day; then squeeze it through a Search into a Barrel, and set it by a Fire: When it has wrought a Fortnight in the Barrel, bung it up, and let it stand till sour enough, which will be according to the Degree of Heat; and in eight or ten Months it is commonly done.

To make Balm Wine.

TO every Chopin of Honey, put three Chopins of Water; boil it on a quick Fire, till one Chopin is boiled away; take Care to keep it closs skimmed, then put it to cool, and put in it a large Handful of Balm, when almost cold, put in it half a Gill of the best Barm, and let it stand till the Head is flat, and done working, which will be in four or five Days, then skim it and strain it through a very fine Search in a Can, but take Care that the Grounds at the Bottom do not mix with it; put it in a Jar, and stop it closs, and when

clear,

clear, bottle it; it will keep feven or eight Years; the older the better. You may make Elder Wine the fame Way of the white Bloffom, but take Care that none of the Stems or green be among them. They both are very wholfome. Meath is made the fame Way, leaving out the Balm and Elder Flowers.

To make Metheglin.

GET fome good ftrong Wort, and to every four Chopins of it, put a Chopin of Honey, boil one Chopin away on a quick Fire, keep it well fkimmed, and when cold, put a Gill of Barm to it, and let it work two or three Days, then put it in your Cafk, a Brandy one is beft for all Wines, if you make a Quantity of them: Get a Bag of Linen, and to every *Englifh* Gallon, put in it two Nutmegs, cut in Quarters a Quarter of an Ounce of Ginger, one Dram of Mace, one of Cloves giofly pounded, put the Bag with thefe in it in the Cafk; bottle it in fix Months, or you may not till twelve.

To make Currant Wine, *white or red.*

TAKE the Currants when they are full ripe, and fqueeze them through a coarfe Cloth, and put to every *Englifh* Gallon of Juice, two Gallons of boiled foft Water, and three Pounds of Sugar; ftir it very well together, then barrel it up, filling up the Barrel every Day, till it has done working, then bung it up clofs, and let it ftand fix Months, and bottle it. Brandy Cafks are beft for all Sorts of made Wine.

To make Gooofeberry Wine.

GATHER the Goofeberries in dry Weather when they are half ripe, bruife them in a Tub with a wooden Mallet or Peftle; then put them in a coarfe Canvas Bag, and prefs out all the Juice; to every *Englifh* Gallon put three Pounds of powdered Sugar, ftir the Sugar in it till it diffolves, then put it in a Cafk, and if you make

but

but a fmall Quantity, put it in a fmall Cafk, for it muft
be full; let it ftand three Weeks, then draw it off, and
pour out the Lees; then put it again into the Cafk and
ftop it clofs, then let it ftand three Months and bottle
it: If you make a large Quantity, let it ftand longer
in the Cask; if you fqueeze a Dozen of bitter Oranges
in it, and put fome of the Rinds pared thin in it, they
will give it a fine Tafte.

Elder-berry *Wine*.

GATHER the Elder berries when they are full
ripe, when it is a very dry Day; then bruife them
with your Hands and ftrain them, then fet the Liquor
by in a Graybeard for twelve Hours to fettle; then
put to every Pint of the Juice. a Pint and a half of
Water; and to every *Englifh* Gallon of this Liquor,
put three Pounds of *Lisbon* Sugar, put it in a Kettle
on the Fire, and when it is almoft boiling clarify it
with the Whites of four Eggs, let it boil an Hour, and
when it is almoft cold, put in it a little ftrong Ale
Barm, and then ton it; and as it works out, fill up
the Veffel with fome of the fame Liquor, in a Month's
Time it will be fit to be bottled; and after it is bot-
led, it will be fit to drink in two Months; but remem
ber that all Liquors muft be fine before they are bot-
led: When it is fine, it will be the better to put in it
a Bottle of Mountain Wine.

To make purging Ale.

TAKE Polipody of the Oak and Senna, of each
two Ounces, of Sarfaparilla an Ounce, Anife feeds and
Carraway Seeds, of each half an Oounce, fix Handfuls
of Scurvy grafs, three of Ground-ivy, one of Agrimony, and one of Maiden-hair, beat all thefe eafily, and
put them in a coarfe Canvas Bag, and hang them in
a Gallon of ftrong Ale that is juft working, and it
will be fit to drink in five or fix Days.

A

To brew strong Ale and small Beer.

BOIL the Water, and put some of the Malt in the Vat, and stir it and the boiling Water very well together, then put in more Malt and more Water mashed pretty thin; then cover the Vat, and let it stand three Hours; then let some of the Wort run, and throw it up again once or twice till it is clear; strew some dry Malt on the Top of the Vat; put your Hops in the Tub that the Wort runs in, and then put them in the brewing Pan on the Fire with the Wort; let it boil till it curdles and then clears; put boiling Water on the Vat by Degrees. Twenty *English* Bushels of Malt will make two Hogsheads of strong Ale, and four Hogsheads of small Beer, but it will take ten Pounds of Hops. This Ale will keep two or three Years; when it is almost as cold as Water, barm it, but strain the Hops out of it when it is warm, and boil them in the small Beer: Let it work three Days, then skim it and barrel it, and when it is done working stop it up close, but keep the Barrel always filling while it is working. *October* or *March* is the best Time to brew.

To make Sydar.

WHEN the Apples are ripe, pull them on a dry Day, and pound them in a Trough with wooden Pounders, then put them in a Hair Bag, and press the Juice out of them; put it in a Brandy or white Wine Cask that is very sweet: put in the Cask some Slices of Apples, and two Penny-worth of Isinglass, stop the Bung close, and bottle it in ten Months.

To make Ratafia.

TAKE three Gallons of Brandy or good Whisky, and blanch and pound half a Pound of bitter Almonds, and put them in the Spirits, with the Rind of Lemons. Let them infuse a Fortnight, then filter off

C c   the

the Spirits, and cork the Bottles clofs you put it in, it is good for any Puddings.

To diftill cold Surfeit Water.

TAKE two Handfuls of Spearmint, two of Balm, one of Angelica, one of Wormwood, one of Carduus, and one of Marigold Flowers; cut them, and put them in Water, then wring them out, and put them in the Still. Keep wet Cloths about it, and a flow Fire under it.

To make Plague Water.

TAKE Rue, Carduus, Balm, Spearmint, Wormwood, Penny royal, Dragon, Marigold Flowers, Angelica and Rofe-mary, of each two Handfuls, cut them fmall, and put them in the Still with Anife-feeds, Carraway, Coriander and fweet Fennel Seeds, then cover them with Spirits, and diftill it off.

To make Shrub.

TAKE five *English* Gallons of Rum, three Chopins of Orange and Lemon Juice, and four Pounds of double refined Sugar; mix all together, but firft pare the Rind of fome of the Lemons and Oranges, and let them infufe in the Rum for fix Hours: Let all run through a Jelly-bag, then cafk it till it is fine, and bottle it.

A very fine Wafh for Ladies that have the Scurvy, or any Rednefs in the Face.

BOIL two Ounces of fine Barley, a Chopin of Water to four Gills, beat two Ounces of Almonds to a Pafte, mixing them with a little of the Barley Water, when cold, warm them, and fqueeze them through a Cloth, then diffolve one Penny-worth of Camphire in a Spoonful of Brandy or any ftrong Spirits. Mix them, and wafh the Face every Night when you are going

ing to Bed: It is the beſt Waſh ever was made for the Face.

The beſt Pomatum for the Lips.

TAKE an Ounce of Spermacete, and mix it with an Ounce of the Oil of bitter Almonds, and a little pounded Cochineal; melt them all together, and ſtrain it through a Cloth in a little Roſe-water, and rub your Lips going to Bed at Night.

To make Eye Water.

GET two Gills of white Roſe-water, put in it the Bigneſs of a Nut of white Vitriol, and the ſame Quantity of the fineſt Loaf Sugar; when it is diſſolved ſhake the Bottle, and waſh the Eyes going to Bed with it, and a ſoft clean Cloth: It is as good an Eye-Water as ever was made.

To make the Sacred Tincture.

PUT in a Mutchkin Bottle five Penny-worth of Hiera Picra, one of Cochineal pounded; then fill the Bottle with Half *Lisbon* Wine, and Half Brandy, tye a Bit of clean Cloth on the Bottle, and put it in a Pan of cold Water, as full that it won't go into the Bottle; put it on a very ſlow Fire, and don't let it boil but ſimmer; then take off the Pan, and let the Bottle ſtand till the Water is cold: It is a very ſafe gentle Phyſick, and good for a Cholick.

To make Stoughton's *Drops.*

INFUSE in a Chopin of *French* Brandy a Penny-worth of Cochineal, a Penny-worth of Snake root, half an Ounce of *Jamaica* Oranges, two Ounces of bitter Orange-peel, one Ounce of Gentian root, two Drachms of *Turkey* Rhubarb, pound the Rhubarb, Cochineal, and *Jamaica* Oranges, ſlice the Gentian; put them near the Fire for two Days in a ſtrong Glaſs Bottle, then put the Bottle in a Pan of cold Water, on a

ſlow

flow Fire: And when it fimmers take off the Pan and when the Water is cold take out the Bottle, let it ftand two Days; then pour off all that is clear, and you may put ftrong Whifkey to the reft, and it will be good for prefent Ufe.

To make Daffy's Elixir.

TAKE a Mutchkin of Brandy, and a Mutchkin of *Lisbon*, infufe in it half an Ounce of Carraway, half an Ounce of Anife-feed, half an Ounce of fweet Fennel-feeds, one Ounce of Hiera-picra, one Ounce of bitter Alloways, two Drachms of Saffron, two Ounces of bitter Orange-peel, and one of Snake-root; let thefe, ly near the Fire for a Fortnight, then put the Bottle in a Pan of cold Water, and when it fimmers take it off; when cold filter it off: You may take two Spoonfuls of it at Night, it is good for a Cholick, and is a gentle Phyfick.

To make the yellow Balfam.

TAKE four Pounds of *May* Butter, and gather in a dry Day a Pound of Elder Flowers, let none of the Stems or Green be in them; mix them with the Butter in a clofs well glazed Can; put it in the Sun by Day, and near the Fire by Night; keep them that Way till the green Broom bloffoms; then get a Pound of the Bloffoms, and mix them very well together, keep them as above for five or fix Weeks; then warm it well, but don't boil it, and wring it all out in a Cloth as well as you can. It is good for any Inflammation, Pain or Stitch, rubbing the Part affected before the Fire with a very little of it, and if inwardly, fwallow five or fix Pills roll'd in Sugar: It is as wholfome and fafe a Thing as ever was taken.

APPEN-

APPENDIX

TO THE

METHOD OF COOKERY.

Apricock Fritters.

GATHER a Dozen and a half of Apricocks juſt beginning to ripen; they muſt not be mellow, nor muſt they be green; this is a very material Circumſtance, for this is a nice Kind of Fritters, and cannot be made in Perfection unleſs the Degree of the Ripeneſs be exactly hit; they are juſt as they ſhould be when they can with ſome Difficulty be opened, and the Stone ſeparated: Having gathered the Apricocks in this State, freſh from the Tree, they are to be prepared for the Fritters in this Manner: Put into a very clean Stew-pan a Quarter of a Pint of *French* Brandy, and a Table Spoonful of the fineſt powdered Sugar; open the Apricocks, take out their Stones, and put the Halves into this Liquor, ſet them for two Hours over a very gentle Stove, ſtirring them from Time to Time with Care not to break them; make a Batter with a large Handful of the fineſt Flour, and as much Mountain Wine as will bring it to a proper Conſiſtence; ſet on another Stew-pan with a large Quantity of Hogs Lard, and when it is thoroughly hot begin to throw in the Fritters made in the following Manner: Throw half an Apricock into the Batter, take it out with as much as hangs about it, and drop it at once into the Lard, ſet a Diſh before the Fire to heat, ſtrew a little fine Sugar over the Bottom of it, and put in the Fritters hot as they come from the Pan; let the Fritters be pretty well browned, which they will be very ſpeedily, and when there are a proper Number in the Diſh, hold a hot Fire Shovel over them for ſome Time, this will glaze them, and then they are to be ſerved up hot; no Sugar is to be put over them. The *French* Apricock Fritters are better than ours, but it is owing to the Goodneſs of

the

the Fruit, they only dip the half Apricocks in Flour, and fry them ; but this has been tried here, and does not anfwer, ours being too watry.

Barley Broth the Scots *Way.*

SET on a large Pot with a Pail full of Water, and let it not be above two thirds filled with this Quantity ; chop a Leg of Beef all to Pieces, breaking the Bones in every Part, and cut into fquare Pieces a good Bunch of found thick Carrots, boil thefe together in the Water, till half is confumed ; towards the End of the Boiling put in a good large Cruft of a brown Loaf toafted and broke to Pieces ; when this is well foftned, and the Gravy is rich, ftrain it off, put it into a fmaller Pot, and add to it half a Pound of *French* Barley, clean eight Heads of Cellery, wafh fome fweet Herbs, and cut two or three good Onions, chop the Cellery to Pieces, and put all in ; let this all boil together twenty Minutes, then pick and wafh a large Fowl, put it into it, and at this Time add fome Parfley chopped fmall, and a few Marigolds , cover it up, and let it boil an Hour longer, then take it off, take out the Fowl, and lay it in the Middle of the Difh , take out the Onion and fweet Herbs, and then pour in the Broth , this is an excellent, rich and well tafted Soup, and is very wholfome.

A boiled Carrot Pudding.

TAKE a Penny white Loaf, and grate it, and grate as much Carrot as Bread, beat feven Eggs, the Whites of three left out, with a little Salt, and a Spoonful of Orange-flower Water, put two large Spoonfuls of Flour, a Pint of Cream, and as much fine Sugar as will fweeten it to your Tafte , laftly, put in a Quarter of a Pound of melted Butter , mix all well together, flour your Bag, and tie it up , let it boil an Hour.

To roaſt a Calf's Liver.

CHUSE a very fine Calf's Liver, and lard it very thick with ſmall Slices of Bacon, faſten it carefully to the Spit, and cover it up with Papers, lay it at a Diſtance before a very good Fire, and obſerve its doing, for no‑thing requires more Time to do nicely; when it is about half done take off the Papers, and bring it a lit‑tle nearer the Fire; and laſt of all, juſt to finiſh it, bring it very near, then ſerve it up in a hot Diſh, with ſome rich Veal Gravy.

To broil Carp.

PREPARE a ſtrong and clear Fire, and warm tho‑roughly a large and clean Gridiron; let the Bars be all hot through, and yet not burning hot upon the Sur‑face, this is the perfect and fine Condition of the Gridiron for nice Uſes; for if it be haſtily heated, the Bars will be hot enough to ſcorch the Things laid on them on their Outſide, and yet cold enough within to chill it, this being made of the Fire and the Gridiron, let the Carp be carefully cleaned, the Fins pulled out, and the Scales perfectly taken off, then rub it over with a Piece of Butter, and ſtrew ſome Salt upon it, lay it on the Gridiron, and watch it very carefully, that it do thoroughly, and not too quick. While the Carp is broiling, the Sauce muſt be prepared thus: Cut to Pieces four Anchovies, half a Cup full of Ca‑pers, and a Quarter of a ſliced Lemon, ſeaſon theſe with Pepper, Salt and Nutmeg, and put them into a Sauce pan with ſome drawn Butter, and a little Vine‑gar, ſend up the Carp when enough, with this Sauce hot.

Sellery in Cream.

CLEAN ſix or eight Heads of Sellery, cut them into Lengths of two or three Inches, and boil them till they are tender; pour away the Water and ſet the Sellery to drain. Put into a Sauce‑pan, half a Pint of Cream,

Cream, and the Yolks of four Eggs beaten up; grate in a little Nutmeg, and sprinkle in a little Basket Salt, then put in the Sellery. Set it over a gentle Fire, let it stew a little, and pour it together into a Dish.

To preserve Cherries with the Stalks and Leaves green.

GATHER some fine Duke Cherries carefully with the Stalks entire, and some Leaves upon them; make some sharp Vinegar boiling hot, dip in the Stalks and Leaves, and scald them well; then lay them on a Sieve that they may dry: Set on a Pipkin or silver Sauce-pan, with two Pounds of the finest Sugar, and a Pint of Water, let this boil up, and it will be a thick Syrup. When this Syrup is boiling hot, dip the Cherries in it with the Stalks and Leaves, and when they are just scalded by it, take them out again, and lay them on a Sieve, then boil up the Syrup to the Height of a Candy, and dip the Cherries into it again, then dry them on Sieves in the same Manner as other Sweet-meats; the Cherries will thus be very fine, and the Leaves will make a pretty Appearance.

A Cowslip Pudding.

PICK the Flowers of a Peck of fresh gathered Cowslips, chop them small, then put them into a marble Mortar, pound them well, and mix with them half a Pound of *Naples* Biscuits, and three Pints of thick and rich Cream, put the Cream in by a little at a Time, but in the End let the whole be well beaten together. Set this all together on the Fire in a large Sauce-pan, mix together three Spoonfuls of Cream, and two Spoonfuls of Rose water, set it by you in a Glass, then break twelve Eggs into a Punch Bowl, beat them up with the Rose water and Cream, and sweeten the whole to your Taste, mix this with the boiling Ingredients in the Sauce pan, and set it off the Fire. Butter a Dish of a proper Size, pour this in, and when it is enough baked, strew some of
the

the fineſt Sugar powdered over it, and ſend it up hot. It is an elegant Pudding.

The beſt Way to pickle Cucumbers.

TAKE the leaſt Cucumbers, rub them well, and put them in a Pot or Barrel, then put in a Round or Lair of Dill or Fennel-ſeed in Branches, and upon that a Lair of Cucumbers, ſo as not to touch one another, ſtrew on them ſome Ginger, Mace and Cloves finely beaten, ſome whole Pepper and a little Salt; then lay in another Lair of each, and fill up the Pot with white Wine or Elder Vinegar. This Pickle ſerves for Grapes or other Things; ſome boil the Vinegar, and pour it on hot, and Elder is beſt done this Way.

Elder Flower Fritters.

GATHER four Bunches of Elder Flowers, juſt as they are beginning to open, for that is the Time of their Perfection, they have juſt then a very fine Smell and a ſpirited Taſte, but afterwards they grow dead and faint; we complain of theſe Flowers having a ſickly Smell, but this is only when they are decaying, when freſh and juſt open they have the ſame Flavour, but it is ſpirited and juſt the contrary of what it is afterwards. The Elder Flowers being thus choſen, break each Bunch into four, regular Parts, lay theſe carefully in a Soup Diſh; break in a Stick of Cinnamon, pour to them a Wine Glaſs of Brandy, and when this has ſtood a Minute or two, add half a Pint of Sack, ſtir the Flowers about in the Liquor, cover them up, and let them ſoak about an Hour, uncovering and ſtirring them about at Times, to ſee how they are kept moiſt, put a Handful of the fineſt Flour into a Stew-pan, add the Yolks of four Eggs beaten, and afterwards their Whites beat up quite to a Foam, add ſome white Wine and a little Salt, and put in the Whites of the Eggs laſt. Let all this be very perfectly and thoroughly mixed, when the

D d   Batter

Batter is thus made, fet on a Quantity of Hog's Lard in a Stew-pan, when it is very hot, fry the Fritters, the Method is this: The Elder Flowers are to be taken out of their Liquor, and put into the Batter, and the Quantity for each Fritter is one of the Bunches of Elder, with as much Batter as agreeably covers it, and hangs well about it. While they are frying, heat the Dish they are to be fent up in, rub a Lemon upon it not cut, and lay in the Fritters as they come out of the Pan, ftrew a little of the fineft Orange-flower Water over them, and ferve them up.

Everlafting Syllabubs.

THIS is a Sort of whipped Syllabub, that will keep a Week or ten Days, and be all the while as good as at firft, and it is a very rich and well tafted Kind. Put in a very large Bowl, half a Pint of Sack, and the fame Quantity of Rhenifh : Squeeze in three large *Seville* Oranges, and add a Pound of the fineft Sugar beaten to Powder ; ftir thefe well together, then grate in the fine upper yellow Part of two large Lemons, ftir it once again together, and then pour in a Quart and half a Pint of rich Cream, beat it about with a Whisk for an Hour, or mill it with a Chocolate Mill, which is the beft Way, and when it is well frothed, put in one Spoonful of Orange-flower Water, beat it up again, and when it is enough, fill the Glaffes with a clean Silver Spoon.

To drefs a Hare the Swifs Way.

SET on a Stew pan with fome ftrong rich Broth, cut a Hare in Quarters, and lard them well with thick Pieces of Bacon, ftrew fome Pepper, Salt and beaten Cloves into the Broth, ftir it together, and then put in the Quarter of the Hare; Cover it up and fet it over a gentle Fire, let it ftew till it is three Parts done, then add a Bottle of red Port Wine, and fome Blades of Mace, cover up the Stew pan again, and fet it over a gentle Fire, to be thoroughly done; when the Hare is near enough make a Sauce thus: Mince the Liver very small, and having saved what Blood you could from the Hare, put these in a Sauce-pan together, dust in a little Flour, and add half a Spoonful of Vinegar; make all these hot together, and while they stand on the Fire, chop a Spoonful of Capers, and cut off the fleshy Part of a Couple of Dozen of Olives, mix all these together in the Sauce pan of Sauce; take out the Hare, and lay the Pieces handsomely and regularly in the Dish. Pour in this Sauce, and serve it up hot.

A Herring Pye.

MAKE a very good Crust, and cover with a Part of it the Bottom of a Dish, scale and gut some fresh Herrings, cut off the Heads and the Fins, wash them very thoroughly, season them with Pepper and Salt, and cut a little Mace very fine, and scatter it over them; lay a Row of Herrings in the Dish, then pare some Apples, and cut them into thin Slices without the Cores, spread a Covering of them over the Herrings, peel some Onions. cut them into Slices and lay them over the Apples in good Quantity, put in some thin Pieces of Butter over the Onions, and then as much Water as will just wet the Fish. Lay on the Crust, and let it be well baked.

To make Mutton Harrico.

CUT a Loin of Mutton into thick Chops, flour them and fry them in a Stew-pan with Butter, till they are browned on both Sides, then pour out the Fat, pour in a small Quantity of boiling Water, and afterwards more, till the Meat freely swims in it, then put in thirty Chesnuts shelled, the Hearts of five Lettices, the Hearts of half a Dozen Onions, two Carrots, and as many Turnips cut in Dice, a Sprig of Thyme and the same of Savoury, two Blades of Mace,

some

ſome Pepper and Bay Salt, and two Cloves; cover it up, and ſet it on a moderate Fire; let it ſtew a couple of Hours, then take off the Fat, and ſend it up together.

Norfolk *Dumplings*.

BEAT up a Couple of Eggs with a little Salt, and by Degrees mix in a Chopin of Milk, then get in as much Flour as will make the Hole into a pretty thick Batter. While this is beating up, let a large and very clean Sauce-pan be ſet on the Fire, three Parts full of Spring Water, when this boils, drop in the Batter in ſuch Quantities at a Time, as will ſerve for a ſmall Dumpling, keep the Water boiling briſkly, and they will be done in three Minutes: Pour off the Water through a Sieve, and lay the Dumpling hot into a Diſh. They are to be ſerved up with a Piece of plain Butter let into each, by cutting a Hole at the Top, they are a very good Kind of Dumpling and coſt ſcarce any Thing but Care; but the greateſt Nicety is required that every Thing be clean, elſe they are ſpoiled.

An Oxford *Pudding.*

CUT as ſmall as poſſible, a Quarter of a Pound of Sewet, grate fine a Quarter of a Pound of Biſcuit, and pick and waſh a Quarter of a Pound of Currants, mix together half a Spoonful of Sugar, a little grated Nutmeg and ſome Salt, a very little of this laſt is ſufficient juſt to take off the Inſipidity: Mix all theſe well together, and ſet them by you, break two Eggs, ſeparate the Yolks, beat them together, and with this mix up the Ingredients into a Paſte, divide this into Lumps of the Bigneſs of a Turkey's Egg, and lay them by you, ſet on a Stew-pan with ſome freſh Butter, fry theſe in it to a fine delicate brown, and take Care that they turn about by the ſhaking of the Pan as they are frying, that they may be thoroughly done, and be

all

all over of a fine light brown; when they are near
enough, melt fome Butter, and add to it a Glafs of
Sack, and a Spoonful of treble refined Sugar beat to
Powder, and fend this up with the Puddings.

A Quaking Pudding.

BREAK fix Eggs, take all the Yolks, and half
the Whites, beat them well up, mix in fome Cream
by Degrees as they are beat, and by Degrees get in a
Pint of it; when thefe are mixed, throw in two Spoonfuls of Rofe-water, and a Tea Spoonful of Orange-
flower Water and a little Salt; grate in fome Nutmeg,
and then add the Crumb of a Half Penny Roll, butter a Cloth very well, and duft a little Flour over it,
then put in the Pudding, and tie it up but not too
clofs, let a Sauce-pan of Water be boiling, and put
it in, keep it boiling brifkly for half an Hour, and it
will be done enough.

To roaft a Saddle of Mutton the French *Way.*

CHUSE a fine fat Saddle or two Loins, cut it together, raife the Skin, and roll it up as far as can be
without breaking it any where, then chop fmall a
good Handful of fweet Herbs and a little Parfley,
bruife fome Pepper, Bay Salt, Mace and a little Nutmeg, mix thefe well with the Hand, then cut into very
thin Slices a Quarter of a Pound of the lean Part of
a good Ham, mix this with the Herbs and Spices, cut
a large Onion very fmall, and fhave very thin fome
Truffles, chop fome Morels, and mix all well together; let the Meat be juft warmed at the Fire,
then lay on thefe Ingredients as even as may be, draw
the Skin over them, and cover the whole with Paper
well butter'd, lay it down to a fteady good Fire, tie it
on the Paper and roaft it in the Manner of Venifon;
when it is enough, take off the Paper, and ftrew upon the Meat fome grated Bread; brown it up well, and
fend it to Table, put a little Shalot under it in the
Difh.

Diſh. This is a high and elegant Diſh in a firſt Courſe.

To ſtuff a Shoulder of Mutton.

THIS is a Diſh to be ſent up with made Gravy, and garniſhed with Horſe-radiſh. The Method of doing it is this : Open a Dozen good large Oiſters, and ſave the Liquor by itſelf, boil three Eggs hard as if for a Sallad; then chop ſmall three Ounces of Beef Sewet, grate to it the ſame Quantity of Bread, rub theſe together when it is about a Quarter done, cut the Skin with a ſharp Knife into Slips, and then finiſh it with a clear good Fire ; ſerve it up with Apple Sauce made with a Blade of Mace, a couple of Cloves, and ſweetened; there ſhould be alſo ſome Muſtard ſent up in a Cup for thoſe who chuſe to eat it that Way.

Soup Sante the Engliſh *Way.*

WE have given in a former Receipt the Method of making Soup Sante according to the *French* Practice ; this which Foreigners call the *Engliſh* Way, makes a Variety, and is a very fine Soup. Make ſome Broth and Gravy in the ſame Manner as is done for the *French* Soup Sante, and for the Receipt, turn back to the Deſcription of that in the former Part of this Work: inſtead of the Herbs uſed in the *French,* put into this a good Quantity of Carrots and Turnips, they muſt be cut into long ſlender Pieces, as big as a Quill and an Inch long, give the Turnips two or three Boils in Water to blanch them, and blanch the Carrots by a longer Boiling. When they are thus prepared, ſtrain off the Water, and put them into two Quarts of the Gravy, add the Cruſt of two *French* Rolls, and boil theſe well together, till the Roots are perfectly tender. To ſend this up to Table, have a Knuckle of Veal boiled, place this in the Middle of the Diſh, and pour the Soup to it, garniſh it with Pieces of Carrot and Pieces of Turnip boiled tender.

A Marrow Pudding, or Whitepot.

SEASON your Marrow with beaten Nutmeg,
Sugar and Salt; then take a Penny Loaf cut in Bits
like Dice, pick some Raisins clean, put in a Dish a
Lair of Raisins, and a Lair of Bread, then a Lair of
Marrow; let them ly in six several Parts; then take a
Pint and a half of Cream, and when it boils put in the
Yolks of four Eggs, with the Whites of two beaten
with a little Nutmeg, Sugar and Salt; stir all well to-
gether, pour it into the Dish upon the Lairs; set it in
the Oven for half an Hour, it being not over hot.

To make Cream Cheese.

TAKE about five Quarts of the Morning Milk, a
Pint and a Half of raw Cream, mix both together, and
run it very hard, then slice it up with a skimming Dish
as thin as you can, and put a fine thin Cloth wet in
a deep large Vat, and fill up the Vat as full as it can
hold, and let it stand till Night; then turn it into another such wet Cloth upon a Pye Plate, so turn it into the Vat again; this do twice a-day till it be hard, a-
bout three Days in the Vat will be enough; then lay
it in a half dry Cloth two or three Days more, according as you see it harden; then put it into Rushes,
pretty thick on both Sides, and in two or three
Days it will be ready for your Use, according as the
Weather is hot or cold, you must change the Rushes
once a day.

A Yorkshire Pudding.

THIS Pudding is to be made when there is a good
Piece of Beef roasting: Beat up four Eggs, mix them
with a Quart of Milk, a little Salt, and as much Flour
as will make it into a middling stiff Batter, a little stif-
fer than is fit for Pancakes; set on a Stew-pan with
some Driping, when it boils pour in the Batter, and
let it bake on the Fire till it is near enough; then turn
a Plate Bottom upwards in the Middle of the Driping-

pan

pan under the Meat, and fet the Stew-pan with the Pudding in it on the Plate; the Fat from the roaft Meat will drop upon it, and the Fire coming freely to the Top of the Pudding, will make it of a fine brown; let it ftand thus till the Meat is done; then drain off the Fat, and fet the Stew-pan on the Fire again, to dry it perfectly well; when this is done, put it into a Difh, cut a Hole in the Middle of it that will hold a China Cup; fill this with Butter melted plain, and fo fend it up to Table. This is an errant *Englifh* Difh, but it is a very good one.

Burgundy Eggs.

PUT into a Mortar two Dozeñ of fweet Almonds blanched; beat thefe to a Mafh, adding a little Milk, then put to them fome bitter Almond Bifcuits grated, and fome Sugar of the fineft Kind in Powder, pound all thefe very well together, break half a Dozen Eggs, beat them up with fome Cream, fome Salt, and a little Orange-flower Water; then put in the pounded Almonds and Bifcuits, ftir all well together, put it into a Sauce-pan, and let it be well done without burning, then pour it into a Difh; duft fome fine powdered Sugar over it, and give it a Colour with a hot Fire-fhovel: Send it up hot, garnifhed with hard Eggs quartered, Yolks and Whites together.

To make a Cuftard Poffet.

TAKE fourteen Eggs, beat them very well, and put to them twelve Spoonfuls of Sack, nine of Ale, and half a Pound of Sugar, fet them upon fome Coals, and warm them, then ftrain them, and fet them on again, and heat them till they begin to thicken, and if you pleafe you may add a little Nutmeg; take one Quart of Cream and boil it, pour it into the Eggs, cover it up, and let it ftand half a Hour, then ferve it up.

Mrs.

Mrs. Banbridge's *Ginger-bread.*

TO two Pounds and a half of Flour add ten Ounces of Butter, half a Pound of Sugar, half an Ounce of Ginger, and a Table Spoonful or two of Carraway Seeds; melt your Butter in a Pound and a half of Treacle, and mix all well together; put it on Tin Plates, and let it be baked very quick, but not ſcorched, when the Oven is pretty cold put it in again to harden.

To preſerve golden, or other Pipins.

TAKE the cleareſt Pipins you can get, and to each Pound of Pipins before they are pared put a Pound of double refined Sugar, and a Pint and a half of Water; ſet the Sugar and Water on the Fire, and when it boils ſkim it; while this is doing pare your Pipins, quarter and core them, and after waſhing them in clear Water, put them into the Syrup on the Fire, and boil them till they are ſoft and clear, adding to them a little Ambergreaſe and Muſk tied up in thin Lawn; take ſome Oranges, peel them, and cut the Peel into little long Bits; boil them in three or four Waters, then in a thin Syrup; when you put up your Pipins, diſtribute theſe Peels among them: You may if you pleaſe uſe Lemon inſtead of Orange-peel.

A boiled Oat-meal Pudding.

BOIL a Pint of Oat meal in three Pints of Milk, and when it is thick like Haſty-pudding, take it off the Fire, waſh and pick a Pound of Currants, and put them between two Cloths to dry, break ſeven Eggs, and beat up all the Yolks, with four of the Whites; ſtir in half a Pound of Butter among the haſty Pudding; add a Glaſs of white Wine to the beaten Eggs, and grate in a Quarter of a Nutmeg, then put them to the reſt, then add the Plumbs, and ſtir all well together, tye it up in a Cloth, and boil it well, then ſend it up with plain melted Butter.

A

A rich Potatoe Pudding.

BOIL two Pounds of fine Potatoes till they are thoroughly done, taking Care they do not break, take them up, and lay them on a Sieve to cool, peel them, put the pure Pulp into a Mortar, and beat it to a Mash, add a Gill of Sack to soften it; then drive it through a Sieve, melt half a Pound of fresh Butter, and mix it with this Pulp of the Potatoes; break ten Eggs, beat up all the Yolks, with three of the Whites, mix these with the Potatoes and Butter, and then add six Ounces of the finest powdered Sugar, and last of all another Gill of Sack, and half a Pint of the richest Cream; grate in a third Part of a Nutmeg, and then stir all very well together, that it may be perfectly mixed. Make some fine Puff Paste, cover the Bottom of a Dish, and raise a Rim round the Sides; pour in this Mixture, and send it to the Oven, let it be baked with a moderate Heat to a fine brown, it is a very elegant baked Pudding: Some add Sweet-meats, and some Currants, but they utterly destroy the true Taste of the other Ingredients.

To pickle Walnuts black.

CHUSE a sufficient Number of Walnuts which are grown to their full Size and are not hardened, this is the exact Time for pickling them this Way, for they have their full Flavour, and yet are soft out of the Stalks, see there be no blemished ones, throw them into a Pan of Pump Water, stir them about, and pour away the Water through a Sieve, mix a Pound of Salt in a Gallon of Water, or make more or less, according to the Quantity of the Walnuts, in the same Proportion, when this is melted, put in the Walnuts, and let them ly two Days, pour away this, and put them into fresh Water, let them ly two Days, then pour that away, put them into fresh Water again, and let them ly three Days, a Week is thus to be taken in the Water soaking, and they will be then ready

dy for the Pickle, put them into a Pot, and fill it a-
bout half; peel a Couple of *Spanish* Onions for a moderate Pot, and stick into each twenty Cloves, put in
a Pint of Mustard Seed, half an Ounce of Mace,
and an Ounce of black Pepper: The common Receipts order all Spice, but it gives them a mawkish
Taste; add six Bay Leaves once broken, and two Sticks
of Horse radish split, when these Ingredients are laid
in, cover them up with more Walnuts, till the Pot is
full, then set on a proper Quantity of very sharp Vinegar, when it boils pour it in, that the Pot may be
quite full, and set a China Plate over it.

To make Elder Wine.

CHOP very small a Quantity of *Malaga* Raisins,
allowing to every Quart of Water a Pound of them;
put the Water and Raisins in an open Vessel, cover it
with a double Cloth, and let it stand in this Manner
nine Days, stirring it very well every Day, then draw
off the Liquor as long as it will run, and after that
press the Raisins to get out the Remainder, mix all
together, and put it up in a Barrel, to every Gallon
of this Liquor add a Pint of the Juice of Elder Berries,
and then stop it up, let it stand six Weeks, then draw
off what is fine into another Vessel, to every Gallon
of this add half a Pound of *Lisbon* Sugar, and let it
stand again till perfectly fine, then draw it off into
Bottles, and let it be kept for Use in a cool Cellar.

To brew Oat Ale, or Barley Ale

THE best Oat Ale in *England* is brewed in
Yorkshire, and the Method they follow is this: Make
a Quantity of Oat-malt with due Care, let it be
made of the white Oat, and dried with Coals, grind
a Quarter of this, and mash it with four and forty
Gallons of cold Water, the softest that can be had, let
it stand all Night, and the next Morning run it off in
a fine small Stream; put into this Liquor two Pounds
of

of fine pale Hops, rubbing them between the Hands, let thefe infufe cold for three Hours, 'and then ftrain the Liquor and tun it, put a moderate Quantity of Yeaft to it, and it will work brifkly for about two Days; when the working is over ftop it up, and let it ftand ten Days, then bottle it off: This makes Oat Ale in the greateft Perfection, but it will not keep long, it drinks very fmooth, brifk and agreeable, and its Colour is fo pale, that it looks like fome Kind of white Wine: When Oat Ale is intended for keeping, it muft be boiled like other Liquors of this Kind, but it is vaftly the lighteft, fineft, and moft elegant Drink this Way. You may do the fame with Barley Malt, it will keep better.

Spirit of Rofemary

GATHER a Pound and a half of the frefh Tops of Rofemary, cut them into a Gallon of clean and fine Melaffes Spirit, and let them ftand all Night, next Day diftill off five Pints with a gentle Heat: This is of the Nature of *Hungary* Water, but not being fo ftrong as that is ufually made, it is better for taking inwardly: A Spoonful is a Dofe, and it is good againft all nervous Complaints.

To make Damfon Wine.

GATHER a large Quantity of Damfons when they are full ripe, prefs them through a Hair-Bag to get out the Juice, and let it ftand an Hour, or two Hours, to fettle, pour it off from the foul Matter at the Bottom, and to every Gallon of the Juice put two Pounds and a half of Sugar beat fine, ftir this all well together, and put it into a Veffel, which muft be filled up to the Top, let it be lightly covered till it has done fermenting, which will be known by the Noife ceafing; then ftop it clofs down, and keep it four Months in the Cafk; after that Time bottle it off, and

it

it will in a little Time be fit for drinking, and will become an excellent and well tasted Wine.

Orange Water.

PEEL a Dozen and half of fine *Seville* Oranges, cut the Rind into small Pieces, and put it into a Still, add to it a Handful of Orange Flowers, two Handfuls of fresh Orange Leaves, and two Gallons and a half of Water; make a Fire under the Still immediately, and distil off a Gallon and a half: This is a very useful Water to be kept in a Family, both for the medicinal Use, and the Service of the Table: It is a very pleasant carminative simple Water, and when there is Occasion to give a Flavour to any of the more elegant Dishes, which is usually ordered to be done by Orange-flower Water, this Orange Water is in many Cases preferable, as in Puddings, and some Creams.

Tar Water.

EVERY one supposes he knows how to cure Tar Water, but it will not be found so on Experience; there is as much Difference between such as is rightly, and such as is injudiciously made, as between Wine and Brandy; the best Proportion I have found upon repeated Trials to be thus: Put a Pound and four Ounces of good Tar into a large earthen Vessel, pour upon it nine Pints of Pump Water; stir it well about with a wooden Ladle, and let it stand four and twenty Hours, then pour the Liquor clear from the Tar, and bottle it up: It may be taken once or twice a-day, a Quarter of a Pint, or more at a Dose; and it is excellent against many Disorders, the Rheumatism, the small Pox, and many others.

Orange Wine.

GET a Dozen Lemons, and fifty *Seville* Oranges, all fine and fresh; pare the Lemons, cut them in Halves, and squeeze them into a Bowl in which there

is

is firſt put two Pounds of fine Sugar broke ſmall; this being ready, ſet on ſix Gallons of Spring Water in a large clean Pot, with a good Fire, put into it twelve Pounds of fine white powdered Sugar, and the Whites of a Dozen of Eggs beat up to a Froth, let it boil an Hour, ſkimming it frequently, let it ſtand till cold, then put into it ſix Spoonfuls of Yeaſt, and the Lemon Juice and Sugar out of the Bowl, firſt ſkimming off the Top; when theſe are mixed well together, pare the Oranges, then ſqueeze in the Juice, and add the yellow Peels, but not the white Part, let it ſtand by covered in a warm Place, and it will quickly work; when it has worked two Days and Nights, put in a Couple of Quarts of good Rheniſh Wine, and then put all together into a Veſſel, let it ſtand then unſtopt till it has done hiſſing, then let it be ſtopt down, and after ſome Time try by pegging whether it be fine, when it is, bottle it off.

Penny-royal *Water.*

GATHER Penny-royal juſt when it is going to flower, cut to Pieces three Pounds of it freſh, and put it immediately into the Still, with ſix Quarts of Water; let it ſtand all Night, and the next Morning diſtill it, put a Piece of brown Paper daubed over with raw Flour and Water Paſte round the Joining of the Head and the Body, and make the Fire briſk, diſtill off a Gallon, this will be excellent Penny-royal Water.

Mint *Water.*

CUT up a Quantity of Speirmint when it has juſt begun to flower, cut to Pieces four Pounds of it, and put it into the Still, with two Gallons of Water, light the Fire directly under it, cloſe the Head on with Flour and Water Paſte, and diſtil off a Gallon, this will be ſtrong, and excellently good.

Aqua . Mirabilis.

BEAT to a grofs Powder an Ounce of Nutmegs, three Quarters of an Ounce of Mace, half an Ounce of Cinnamon, and a Quarter of an Ounce of Cloves, put them into a Still, with a Gallon of Melaffes Spirit, and three Quarts of Water, and immediately make the Fire diftil off three Quarts and a Pint, and add three Pints of Water, with a Quarter of a Pound of fine Sugar diffolved in it, this is a fine Cordial, the Name is *Latin*, and fignifies *The wonderful Water*, and it very well deferves that Title.

To make Roffoly the Italian *Way.*

GATHER frefh Damask Rofes, Orange Flowers, Jeffamy Flowers, Cloves, and Gilly Flowers, pick them clean, fet on fome Water to boil, when it has boiled well, let it ftand to cool a little, put thefe clean Flowers into a China Bafon, pour the Water upon them when it is no hotter than to bear the Finger in it, then cover it up, and let it ftand three Hours, gently pour all into a fine Linen Bag, and let the Water run off without fqueezing the Flowers, to a Pint of this Water add a Quart of fine Melaffes Spirit, and half a Pint of ftrong Cinnamon Water, add three Tea Spoonfuls of Effence of Ambergreafe, and ftir all well together. This is the true Roffoly.

Orange Wine with Raifins.

FEW made Wines are the Produce of this Seafon for Want of Fruits, but we fhall inftance this as one fit for the Seafon Put eight Gallons of Water in a fmall Copper, and boil away a third Part of it, then fet it to cool a little, pick thirty Pounds of Malaga Raifins, chop them very fmall, and fet them in Readinefs, chufe twenty very large and fine *Seville* Oranges, pare half of them very thin, put the Peels to the Raifins in a large Tub, and pour upon them five Gallons of Water tolerably hot, let thefe ftand
together

together five Days, stirring it well once or twice a Day, then let it be strained through a Hair-sieve, pressing it pretty briskly; put this Liquor in a Runlet, and put into it the Rinds of the other ten Oranges cut thin, after this press out the Juice of the twenty Oranges and boil it up with a Pound of fine Sugar, add this to the Liquor, and stir it well together, then stop it up close, and set it by for two Months, after which bottle it up.

Plague *Water*.

CUT to small Pieces half a Pound of fresh Sage, a Quarter of a Pound of dry *Roman* Wormwood, three Quarters of a Pound of fresh Rue, half a Pound of dried Mint, and four Ounces of fresh Rosemary; add to these an Ounce and a half of fresh Angelica Root, and two Ounces of *Virginian* Snake-root, put these into the Bucket headed Still, with a Gallon of Melasses Spirit, and a Gallon of Water, let them stand all Night, and the next Morning distill off three Quarts, add to this two Quarts of Water, with a Quarter of a Pound of fine Sugar dissolved in it. This is an easy Receipt, and makes the Water very fine.

Birch Wine.

FIX upon a tall strait Birch Tree, and watch when the Buds look plump and forward, this is about the Middle of *March*, bore a deep Hole in the Trunk of the Tree slanting downwards, stick in a Chip, and set a Vessel under to catch what runs, do this to several other thriving Trees, and save and mix all the Juice together, it will be thin, clear and well tasted, set this Juice over the Fire in a large preserving Pan, skim it as any Thing rises, and when it is warm, put into every Gallon of the Liquor, four Pounds and a half of Lump Sugar broke to Pieces, that it may melt the easier; throw in at the same Time the Peel of a good Lemon fresh cut, boil it half an Hour, and keep skimming as any Thing rises, pour it off into a clean
small

fmall Tub, toaft half a Pound of Loaf, fpread it well
over with Yeaft, and put this into the Liquor when
it is almoft cold; let it ftand thus five Days, ftirring
it about frequently, and at the End of that Time, get
a Barrel ready that will hold it and no more; burn a
Brimftone Match in this, and then pour in the Wine,
lay the Bung lightly in the Hole till it has done working, then ftop it faft in, and pour fome melted Pitch
over it. Let it ftand three Months in the Cafk, and
then bottle it off.

Angelica Water.

TAKE of the Leaves of Angelica four Pounds,
Annife-feeds three Ounces, Coriander and Carraway-
feeds of each four Ounces; cut the Leaves fmall, and
bruife the Seeds carefully together in a Mortar, put
them into the Still with fix Gallons of white Wine,
and let them ftand all Night, the next Morning put in
three Drams of Zedoary Root cut into very thin Slices,
and a Handful of frefh Clove Gilly flowers, the fame
Quantity of Sage-flowers, and the fame Quantity of
the Tops and Leaves of fweet Marjoram, when all
are in, ftir them well up with a Stick, and then put
on the Head of the Still, clofe it with a Paper wet-
ted with Flour and Water Pafte, and then diftill off
the Liquor; the Quantity to be drawn off is three
Gallons; it is excellent in Diforders of the Stomach
and Head, and againft Wind.

Malaga Raifin Wine.

WE propofe here to lay down the eafy and familiar
Way of making this excellent Wine: Chufe fome fine
whole and fweet Malaga Raifins, put a Quarter of a
hundred of them into a fmall Cafk, and pour upon them
feven Gallons of cold Spring Water, cover this flightly
and fet it in a warm Place, let it keep there fome
Weeks;

Weeks; the Water will swell and burst the Raisins, and the whole will ferment, there will be a hissing Noise and a Froth at the Top; when this is over, the Liquor is to be managed as we have before directed, keeping it a proper Time in the Cask, and then bottling it, and it is a pleasant wholsome Wine, which may be improved in Colour, by being tinged to a light yellow with Saffron Paper. The Time of the Wine's standing should be about five Months, it is then to be drawn off into another Vessel, and in three Months more it will be fine and fit for bottling, or it may be drawn off in a Decanter as used, the best Time to put in the Saffron Paper is, when it is drawn into the second Cask, and a small Quantity is sufficient. This not only gives an agreeable Colour like Mountain, instead of the watery Whiteness of the common Raisin Wine, but it helps the fining of the Wine, and gives it a pleasant Flavour. One Caution must be given in this Case, which is to take particular Care the Saffron Papers are good and genuine; they should be bought of the People who cure the Saffron, they have a good Smell when genuine, and a deep Orange red Colour, too many counterfeit them, and those will give the Wine an ill Taste. The right Saffron Papers are what cover the Cakes of Saffron in the drying, but the others are stained with Turmerick.

Compound Annise-seed Water.

BRUISE in a large Mortar half a Pound of Annise-seeds, and the same Quantity of Angelica Seeds dried, put them into a Still, pour on them a Gallon of Proof Spirit and three Quarts of Water, fix on the Head, make a brisk Fire, and distill off three Quarts and three Quarters of a Pint, add a Pint and a Quarter of Water, and set it by for Use. This has all the Virtues of common Annise-seed Water, in dispelling Wind, and is besides a great Cordial, it is also much pleasanter than the common Annise-seed: No

Water

Water is better than this againſt the Cholick, and any Sickneſs ariſing from Victuals diſagreeing with the Stomach; none better when going into a bad Air, a Tea Spoonful of this Water put into half a Pint of an Infant's Victuals, is very good againſt the Wind with which thoſe tender Creatures are frequently tormented.

Cherry Wine.

GATHER ſome ripe Cherries, and if there be any to ſpare of the firſt ripe Kinds, none are ſo proper, for there is not any Cherry whatever that has a richer Juice for Wine, than the *May* Duke; take off the Stalks, and bruiſe the Cherries in a Hair-ſieve, ſo as to get out the Juice without bruiſing the Stones, meaſure the clear Juice, and to every Gallon of it, put two Pounds of Lump Sugar beat to Powder, ſtir this well together, and have a clean Veſſel that will juſt hold the Quantity, let it be lightly covered and worked, watch it at Times, and when it does not make any more Noiſe, ſtop it cloſe up, let it ſtand thus for three Months, and then bottle it off and ſet it in a good Cellar. It is a very agreeable weak Wine.

To make Cowſlip or Primroſe Wine.

TAKE three Gallons of fair Water, put into it ſix Pounds of the fineſt Sugar, boil them together half an Hour and more, taking off the Scum carefully as it riſes, then pour it into a Pan or Tub to cool, when it is almoſt cold, take a Spoonful of Ale Yeaſt, and beat it well with ſix Ounces of Syrup of Lemon, mix this with the Liquor by toſſing it up and down, then take a Gallon of picked Cowſlips or Primroſes, bruiſe them in a marble Mortar, and put them into the Liquor, let them work together two or three Days, then ſtrain it off and put it into a Veſſel that is juſt fit for it, two or three Days after ſtop it cloſe, and three

Weeks

Weeks or a Month after that bottle it off, putting a Lump of Sugar into every Bottle. If it is well cork. ed, it will keep a Year.

To make a Cordial Water.

TAKE Rosemary, sweet Balm, red Sage, Rue, dried Mint, Myrrh, Mugwort and Angelica, of each half a Pound, Angelica Roots, three Ounces, Dittany, a Quarter of a Pound; Carduus, Betony, Scabius, Pimpernel, Agrimony, Tormentil Roots and Celandine, of each half a Pound; Gentian Roots, two Ounces, and Rosa Solis two Quarts; steep all these Herbs and Roots, being first cut small and bruised, twelve Hours in five Gallons of white Wine, and distill it off quickly in two cold Stills.

Another Way to make Cowslip, or Clove gilly-flower Wine.

TAKE a Gallon of Water to a Quart of Honey; let your Water boil before you put the Honey in, then let it boil again, and skim it carefully; after it has boiled some Time take it off, and let it stand to cool, work it as in the former Receipt, and when it has half done working, put in the Cowslips or Gilly-flowers, if Gilly-flowers, they must be dried two or three Days before you put them in; when it has stood a little, turn it up in a Vessel, and let it remain a Month before you bottle it off: This is admirable Drink, without the Flowers, and will keep half a Year, but if you would have it keep a Year, put two Quarts of Honey to a Gallon of Water.

Currant Wine.

CHUSE a dry Day for gathering the Fruit; gather it full ripe, strip the Berries clean from the Stalks, and put them into a large earthen Pan, bruise them with the Pestle of a Marble Mortar till they be all thoroughly broken, let them stand four and twenty

Hours

Hours in the Pan; in this Time they will ferment, and the Juice which was thick will by that Means grow thin; then pour the whole into a Hair Sieve set over a Pan large enough to hold the Juice; it will run freely through, and is not to be squeezed or forced at all: The Juice being thus obtained, to every Gallon of it put three Pounds and a half of *Lisbon* Sugar, stir it well together, and put it into the Vessel; if you have six Gallons of it put in a Quart of Brandy, and the same Proportion to any greater or smaller Quantity; the Vessel should be full, and it should stand six Weeks, then let it be examined, and if it be fine bottle it off; if it be not fine enough for bottling, let it be drawn from the Lees into another Cask, and from that bottle it, after it has stood a Fortnight, for in that Time it will generally grow thoroughly fine and clear.

NECES.

NECESSARY DIRECTIONS,

Whereby the Reader may eafily attain the ufeful Art of CARVING.

To cut up a Turkey.

RAISE the Leg, open the Joint, but be fure not to take off the Leg; lace down both Sides of the Breaft, and open the Pinion of the Breaft, but do not take it off; raife the Merry-thought between the Breaft-bone and the Top, raife the Brawn, and turn it outward on both Sides, but be careful not to cut it off, nor break it; divide the Wing pinions from the Joint next the Body, and ftick each Pinion where the Brawn was turned out; cut off the fharp End of the Pinion, and the Middle Piece will fit the Place exactly. A Buftard, Capon, or Pheafant, is cut up in the fame Manner.

To rear a Goofe.

CUT off both Legs in the Manner of Shoulders of Lamb; take off the Belly-piece clofe to the Extremity of the Breaft, lace the Goofe down both Sides of the Breaft, about half an Inch from the fharp Bone, divide the Pinions, and the Flefh firft laced with your Knife, which muft be raifed from the Bone, and taken off with the Pinion from the Body, then cut up the Merry-thought, and cut another Slice from the Breaft-bone, quite through, laftly, turn up the Carcafe, cutting it afunder, the Back above the Loin bones.

To unbrace a Mallard or Duck.

FIRST, raife the Pinions and Legs, but cut them not off; then raife the Merry-thought from the Breaft, and lace it down both Sides with your Knife.

To unlace a Coney.

THE Back muſt be turned downward, and the Apron divided from the Belly; this done, ſlip in your Knife between the Kidneys, looſening the Fleſh on each Side; then turn the Belly, cut the Back croſs-ways between the Wings, draw your Knife down both Sides of the Back-bone, dividing the Sides and Leg from the Back. Obſerve not to pull the Leg too violently from the Bone, when you open the Side, but with great Exactneſs lay open the Sides from the Scut to the Shoulder, and then put the Legs together.

To wing a Partridge or Quail.

AFTER having raiſed the Legs and Wings, uſe Salt, and powdered Ginger, for Sauce.

To allay a Pheaſant or Teal.

THIS differs in nothing from the foregoing, but that you muſt uſe Salt only for Sauce.

To diſmember a Hern.

CUT off the Legs, lace the Breaſt down each Side, and open the Breaſt Pinion, without cutting it off; raiſe the Merry-thought between the Breaſt-bone and the Top of it; then raiſe the Brawn, turning it out-ward on both Sides, but break it not, nor cut it off; ſever the Wing pinion from the Joint neareſt the Bo-dy, ſticking the Pinions in the Place where the Brawn was. Remember to cut off the ſharp End of the Pi-nion, and ſupply the Place with the Middle Piece. In this Manner ſome People cut up a Capon or Phea-ſant, and likewiſe a Bittern, uſing no Sauce but Salt.

To thigh a Woodcock.

THE Legs and Wings muſt be raiſed in the Man-ner of a Fowl, only open the Head for the Brains. And ſo you thigh Curlews, Plover or Snipe, uſing no Sauce but Salt.

To

To display a Crane.

AFTER his Legs are unfolded, cut off the Wings; take them up, and fauce them with powder'd Ginger, Vinegar, Salt, and Muftard.

To lift a Swan.

SLIT it fairly down the Middle of the Breaft, clean through the Back, from the Néck to the Rump; divide it in two Parts, neither breaking or tearing the Flefh; then lay the Halves in a Charger, the flit Sides downwards; throw Salt upon it, and fet it again on the Table. The Sauce muft be Chaldron, ferved up in Saucers.

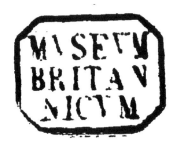

F I N I S.

9 781170 606292